PENGUIN BOOKS

HELPING YOUR HAN.

Janet Carr read psychology at Reading University and, after
gaining a diploma in clinical psychology at the Maudsley Hospital, worked in mental hospitals and child guidance clinics.
She carried out a longitudinal study of children with Down's
syndrome, which led to a Ph.D. at the London University
Institute of Education.

From 1970 to 1978 she was a lecturer in the Psychology
Department of the London University Institute of Psychiatry
and Senior Psychologist at Hilda Lewis House, a hospital-based
unit for the assessment and treatment of severely learning-
disabled children. She became involved in the teaching of behavioural methods and as a result has run numerous courses, for
professionals and parents, both in this country and in Sweden,
Australia and Iceland.

Janet Carr retired from St George's Hospital Medical School,
London, in 1992. Her publications include *Young Children with
Down's Syndrome*, *Behaviour Modification for People with Mental
Handicaps* (co-edited with William Yule), *Working Towards Inde-
pendence* (with Suzanne Collins) and *Down's Syndrome: Children
Growing Up*.

Janet Carr

Helping Your Handicapped Child

SECOND EDITION

With a new Foreword by Professor Peter Mittler

PENGUIN BOOKS

PENGUIN BOOKS

Published by the Penguin Group
Penguin Books Ltd, 27 Wrights Lane, London w8 5tz, England
Penguin Books USA Inc., 375 Hudson Street, New York, New York 10014, USA
Penguin Books Australia Ltd, Ringwood, Victoria, Australia
Penguin Books Canada Ltd, 10 Alcorn Avenue, Toronto, Ontario, Canada m4v 3b2
Penguin Books (NZ) Ltd, 182–190 Wairau Road, Auckland 10, New Zealand

Penguin Books Ltd, Registered Offices: Harmondsworth, Middlesex, England

First published 1980
Second edition 1995
10 9 8 7 6 5 4 3 2 1

Filmset by Datix International Limited, Bungay, Suffolk
Printed in England by Clays, Ltd, St Ives plc
Set in 10/12 pt Monophoto Imprint

To Karl, Katy, Paul, Ruth, Chris, Carla, Jane, Lisa, Howard and Graeme: and to all the other children who go to Dysart School, Kingston-upon-Thames, for whose parents this book was originally written

Contents

Foreword

That parents can be effective and successful teachers of their own children should occasion neither surprise nor congratulation, since they have been doing it for millennia. With the passage of time, parents have come to share the task with teachers for a few years, but more recently teachers have begun to call on the experience of parents in coming to a better understanding of children's preferences and learning styles. The task for the twenty-first century is to forge a new partnership between teachers and parents in order to pool their experience so that they can work together in the interests of children.

The need for partnership and collaboration between professionals and parents is particularly important where children have learning difficulties or disabilities. Their parents do not all have access to professionals with experience of working with children with disabilities. The child may not yet be old enough to go to school; the professionals may be well-meaning but relatively inexperienced or only partly trained to work in this field, or they may be more competent and confident in working with children than in sharing their skills with parents.

This book is aimed at all parents who have a child with a learning disability. It provides a lifeline for new parents who are daily facing the challenge of fostering their child's learning and development alone and without support. It offers sound advice and practical suggestions for other parents who are looking for new ideas and approaches to helping their child. It sets out some basic principles of teaching and learning and shows how they can be applied in everyday settings in the home.

The book does not provide a set of ready-made exercises and prescriptions, or guarantee growth and development. Nor does it suggest that teaching has to be in the form of one to one sessions which may lead to tears and frustration all round. Parents can take advantage of natural opportunities for teaching and learning which occur in the ordinary routines of the household. Each family will have to decide for themselves how much they can do and how much teaching is in the interests of their child. Nor should it be assumed that all the teaching is done be the mother; all members of the family and the household can make a joint as well as a distinctive contribution without subjecting the child with a learning disability to constant pressure to learn something new.

The book should provide a source of encouragement and support and perhaps a sense of solidarity with the many parents who have 'been there' before them.

Professor Peter Mittler, CBE, Ph.D.
University of Manchester

Preface to the Second Edition

Since this book first appeared in 1980 there have been changes in many areas of learning disability. In this edition I have tried to reflect these changes by including some of the new approaches that have been developed and by updating the terminology. So in this latter respect, instead of 'mental handicap' (which was in general use in 1980) we use the term, now widely accepted in this country, 'learning disability'. The exception to this is the title, which in the interest of continuity has been kept as it was originally.

In the 1980 edition, when referring to 'the child', when this meant children in general rather than any particular child under discussion, the masculine pronoun was used; in this edition, in order to be scrupulously even-handed, it is the turn of the feminine gender, and 'the child' is now referred to as 'she'.

Acknowledgements

I owe a great deal to the late Professor Jack Tizard and to Dr Elizabeth Newson for their helpful and constructive criticism of the manuscript; to Glyn Murphy who wrote the first draft of the chapter on play besides reading and commenting on the rest of the manuscript; to my family who put up with me while I was writing it and who are on two or three occasions pictured within; and finally to the Parents' Group at Dysart School, Kingston-upon-Thames, without whom this book would not have been written.

Second Edition

I am deeply grateful to Patricia Howlin, who has contributed an enormous amount of time, energy and expertise to the revision of this book; to all the other people who ensured that the revised edition saw the light of day; and to Eleo Gordon of Penguin Books, the most helpful and encouraging editor I have so far encountered.

1. About This Book

To most people, the news that their child has learning disabilities comes as a tremendous blow.

As a parent has said, 'Being told for the first time that one's child is retarded may well be the most severe shock that one may experience in a normal lifetime full of trying experiences'.*

When the first shock is past, most parents want to know what they can do for their child. How can we help her? How should we teach her? What should we teach her? What will she be able to learn? How can we give her the best possible opportunities so that, even if her abilities are limited, she can make the most of them?

Until recently there were not many answers to these questions, and the answers that there were seldom came the way of parents. With little help or guidance available, many parents fell back on the only rule they knew: bring the child up as normal. (Indeed this not specially helpful advice has often been handed out by professionals.) For some children this approach suffices: they learn reasonably well what they need to learn and their parents have few problems with them. But with others, the ordinary ways of bringing up ordinary children are less successful. Many children with learning disabilities do have special difficulties. In particular, although most children pick up a great deal from their surroundings and from watching what other people do, children with learning disabilities often cannot. Because of this they may seem unteachable and may be written off as incapable of learning. In fact they *can* learn, but may need special teaching, and special ways of teaching, to do

* 'A parent discusses initial counselling', H. Raech, *Mental Retardation*, vol. 2, 1966, pp. 25–6.

so. This book is concerned with one such way of teaching, behavioural methods.

What are behavioural methods?

Behavioural methods consist of a set of ways aimed at changing what people do – their behaviour. By 'behaviour' I mean anything that the child does; a wave of the hand, a kiss, a kick, jumping into a puddle, saying 'bye-bye'. This isn't quite the way the word is used ordinarily, when it tends to cover a longer period of time, as in 'Tommy behaved well today'. This slightly specialized use of a word is not unusual in discussing technical matters and we shall come across it again with other words in the book, but as it is always pretty clear what is meant it need not bother anyone. However, perhaps I should stress that the behaviour I am talking about is not, primarily, a matter of what the child may be thinking or feeling (though, of course, this too is important), but of observable things – what she *does*. The methods I will be discussing here are very practical.

Behavioural methods are based on the idea that what we do is influenced by what happens immediately afterwards. If, when we do something, what happens next is something pleasant, we will be likely to want to do that thing again; if it is not, we will be less likely to want to do it again.

So, when we want a child to learn, we look very carefully to see what she particularly enjoys; then we try to make sure that she gets one of these enjoyable things when she does what we want her to do, and that she does not get it when she does something we would rather she did not. Suppose, for example, she loved praise and attention, and suppose we wanted to teach her to put things in a box and not to throw them round the room; then we would make sure that when she put something in the box she got lots of praise, while if she threw things around she did not get any attention at all – we might even look away from her, apparently bored.

Behavioural methods also lay stress on ways of teaching that are adapted to suit the child. When we have decided on something we want the child to learn – say, using a spoon or putting on a sock – if we find it is too difficult for her, then we break the task up into smaller bits and teach them to her one at a time. As each bit is learned it is joined up to the next, until finally she succeeds in the whole task that seemed so impossible at the beginning. We may need to observe progress and record it, since over a short period change may not be easily perceived. All this is less difficult than it sounds, and in later chapters there is plenty of practical guidance on how to go about it.

By this time some readers may be getting a bit uneasy. What about the ethics of all this? Isn't it a bit like brainwashing? Maybe it would be all right with non-disabled children, but is it right to use it with someone as vulnerable as a learning-disabled child? I would like to discuss this uncertainty both because of the very real fear it expresses and because in showing the fears are mistaken we shall see more clearly what behavioural methods aim to achieve.

One of the most important things they set out to do is to help the child understand what we are trying to convey to her by simplifying the messages we give her. Normal communication is a complicated process, but with most children this simplification is not usually necessary: they are able to take in and respond to the jumble of signals we give out by gesture, facial expression, emphasis of speech, and to sort out what matters and what doesn't. For the child with learning disabilities this may be just too difficult, and she may fail to respond not because she *can't* but because she doesn't *understand* what we want her to do. Behavioural methods help us to sort out our messages, to make them simpler and clearer, so that the child has a better chance of understanding and responding.

Secondly, behavioural methods are a way of opening up to the child a whole range of interesting and useful experiences. Most children can be introduced to these in words; we can tell them about new things, or explain why we think it is a good idea for them to learn this or that. They may or may not be convinced by our arguments, but at least they know about them and can decide for themselves. The child with learning disabilities, however, often has a special problem with language. She may be unable to understand what we say, to grasp an idea, to think about it and make up her mind whether or not she will give it a try. By using behavioural methods we can introduce the child to things she might otherwise never experience – riding a bike, putting on records, playing with toys. When she has tried out these new experiences then she can decide whether or not they are for her.

I think it's important to emphasize this – the potential enrichment of the child's life, and the limitations of the methods. By using them we can help the child to understand what we want her to do and to enjoy doing it, but even if we wanted to we cannot force behaviours from her. What we can do is to make them available to her, enable her to choose to do them. The aim is to free her as far as possible from the restrictions of her disability, to help her become more independent and able to make decisions for herself. Behavioural methods *can* help.

I have stressed that these methods are especially important in teaching children with learning disabilities but they are used a great deal, too, with other children, to help them learn, pay attention in class, become toilet-trained, get over temper tantrums and sleeping difficulties, and hundreds of other ordinary and not-so-ordinary childhood problems. I myself used one of these methods, a token programme (see chapter 4), to help my son work for an exam he wanted to pass. Many parents who have used these methods in order to help a child with disabilities have gone on to use them with their other children too. There is nothing strange about behavioural methods; they are just a very careful way of teaching.

Some people may feel that they are being asked to behave in a rather artificial and unspontaneous way, but this may be necessary only for the particular problem they are tackling;

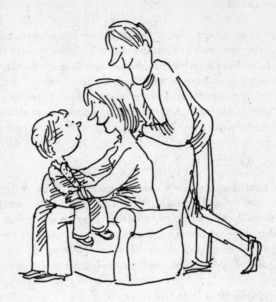

otherwise life goes on as normal, as loving and caring, friendly or cross, organized or disorganized as ever it was. Moreover, once the problem is behind them, most parents will be able to slide gently back to more normal ways of behaving, but at the same time they know that if a new problem arises they can return to behavioural methods to help them over this new hump; while some parents may find that certain methods become more or less second nature to them and will use them more often than not – paying attention to the good things the child does, perhaps, or affecting indifference to tiresome behaviour. Others will not want to use behavioural methods at all, some may use them quite briefly, some for a bit longer. For those who think behavioural methods might help them, this book offers some guidelines on how to go about it.

Getting started

The book is in two parts. In Part 1, which is about ways of teaching, chapters 2–7 are concerned with behavioural methods in general. In Part 2, which is about teaching particular things, chapters 8–12 are about some skills which parents often want their children to learn and chapter 13 about helping children get over fears. Finally, chapter 14 has some suggestions about continuing the work.

What to teach?

Behavioural methods are ways of teaching: they tell you *how* to teach, not *what* to teach. You can teach your child what you think she needs to learn, whether it is an everyday activity like feeding or dressing (described in chapters 8–11) or whether it is something quite different. Whatever you decide on you can, if you want, use behavioural methods in your teaching.

Some people find it helps to make a list of the things they would most immediately like the child to learn to do and not to do, and put them in order of priority. As a rule it is a good idea to work on only one or two to begin with – too many at a time can be muddling – and to work on a positive, learning-to-do, project at the same time as a learning-not-to-do one. There are usually plenty of positive things to teach, and it is enjoyable for everybody to see the child making progress in something new.

How much time each day?

How much time you will need to spend on teaching depends, of course, on the kind of problem you are tackling and on the other demands on your life. As a rough guide other parents have usually spent between five minutes and half an hour a day. With a very distractible child five minutes may well be enough. Little-and-often is a good general rule: two sessions of five minutes are probably better than one of ten.

Some behaviour, such as throwing things about, can't be dealt with in a single session each day at a particular time. You just have to deal with it when it happens. If it doesn't happen too often – only once or twice a day – you may be able to deal with it any time it occurs. Similarly, if the best treatment is a fairly easy one to use, like time-out from your attention (turning your head away, or in some way refusing to pay attention to what the child is doing), you may be able to use it every time the behaviour occurs. If, on the other hand, the child's bad behaviour happens very often, and you have decided that you should use a treatment method like restraint (holding the child quite still for a short time) which demands your full attention, so that it is impossible to do if the behaviour happens just when you are pouring tea for a nervous aunt or dealing with a pan of boiling fat, then you may at first decide to deal with it only in certain situations.

Suppose, for instance, the bad behaviour was throwing things and you had decided to use restraint. You might decide that first thing in the morning is too hectic a time for you to do this, but you could manage it between 4 and 6 p.m., after your child gets home from school and before you start on the evening meal. If you kept careful records over the weeks of how often the child threw things during the 4–6 treatment time, you would be able to see whether the method you were using was a useful one – that is, whether the child was throwing things around less often. If this were the case you might find it possible to extend the treatment into a little more of the day – success works wonders.

The important point is that the methods described in this book are meant to help your child and you, not to make life difficult. What you decide to do must be possible, given your situation. You too have a life, so has your partner, and so have your other children. I am not asking you to spend every available minute with your child, to dedicate yourself body and soul to her. She might indeed learn a great deal by such intensive teaching, but you might end up so exhausted that you had to give up teaching her altogether, so the benefit would be short-lived. Many teachers (and of course I include parents in this term) have found that a learning-disabled child can gain a great deal from a short amount of teaching each day geared to her special needs. I hope also that in reading this book you will discover ways of casual, informal teaching and of responding to her (for instance by noticing and appreciating tiny bits of 'good' behaviour) that can go on for most of her waking hours without making undue demands on your time and energy.

Brothers and sisters

Parents with other children may wonder about the effect on them of all this work with the child with learning disabilities. Of course, I hope the work will not take up so much time that the other children feel badly neglected. All the same this is a question to think about. In general there are three main things you can do:

1. Give time to the other children on their own. This is fairly obvious. Most parents are aware of the need to give some time to the other children and do their best to fulfil it.

2. Give the other children a programme of their own. This is on the whole most suitable for young brothers and sisters. They may be included because their parents see that these children, too, can benefit from behavioural methods – one sister had a programme to help her keep her bedroom tidy and another little brother a similar (very successful) one to help him not to wet his bed. Or the other children can be included just so that they do not feel left out. When Hugh was going to be given sweets for washing and dressing himself in the morning his mother was asked whether she thought this would cause any upset with his very small sister. 'Oh, no,' she replied, 'that won't be any trouble. She can get sweets for putting her toys away, or helping me around the house. We'll think of something. We'll make sure she doesn't lose out.'

3. Include the other children in the teaching. This is where older brothers and sisters come in. Many parents feel, rightly, that they do not want to overburden their other children with responsibility for the disabled child. But brothers and sisters are often glad to do something positive and can enjoy helping to observe behaviour or run teaching sessions (even if, like one mother, their parents boggle at their being involved in dealing with the 'bad' behaviour; 'I'm not having her bossing Tess about'). If a brother or sister wants to do some of the teaching it is a good idea for him or her to do one or two sessions alongside the parent, to make sure that things are being done in the same way, observations made, and rewards given.

Brothers and sisters can be very good teachers and can get a great deal of satisfaction from teaching and helping a learning-disabled sibling.

How long will it take the child to learn?

This can vary a lot from problem to problem and child to child. Sometimes a child can take months to learn something that looks quite simple, like matching colours; sometimes a really daunting problem, like putting uneatable things in the mouth, can be overcome quite quickly. One child took nearly a year to learn not to wet her bed, another became dry over a period of a few weeks. There is no real way of telling in advance how long it will take to overcome a problem completely, but progress along the way is very encouraging.

What, though, if things don't go well, or go very slowly?

When things don't go well

It is helpful to realize that irregular progress in this kind of teaching is quite common. Several good sessions can be followed by a terrible session, even two or three sessions together. The progress chart, instead of being a smooth steady upward slope like a telegraph wire going up a mountainside, resembles instead the Atlantic in a force eight gale, climbing up and plunging down.

There may be some reason for the child's dropping back – she may be unwell, or some change in her surroundings, like a new teacher at school, may be disturbing her. If you are fairly sure you are working along the right lines it may be best simply to persist with the programme. Evan, who was learning not to wet his bed, had kept it dry up till 9.30 in the evening six nights out of seven for about nine weeks. All of a sudden, for no apparent reason, the dry beds dropped to five and then wavered about between five and two for five more weeks. His mother persisted and Evan went up to six dry beds and then, again for no special reason that she could see, suddenly, for the first time in the nine years of his life, began to be dry not only through the evening, but also frequently at 7 in the morning.

Here persistence paid off, so we should not give up too easily. But what if things continue to go badly? First of all, don't get discouraged. Don't think:

'It's my fault (I'm not able to do this sort of thing well enough).'

'It's her fault (she's too disabled/stubborn/wicked ever to learn).'

'Behavioural methods don't work (just like all the other methods).'

What you need here is a change of tactics. And to achieve this you should discuss your problems with someone. Perhaps another member of the family would help – a son or daughter, if both parents are already involved, or a grandparent, aunt or uncle; or perhaps a friendly neighbour or interested friend. One of them might discuss the problems with you, read over the relevant parts of this book and help you plan afresh. What one person does not understand the other may find reasonably clear and be able to explain. When one is flagging the other may be able to inspire fresh enthusiasm.

The two-heads-are-better-than-one approach paid off for this family: 'We wanted to teach Tess not to put everything in her mouth. We wondered whether we should use time-out for her, but I couldn't see how you were supposed to do it. Then my husband and I read through that part of the chapter together and talked it over, and then I found I could understand it and we used it with Tess. It worked too – she hardly ever puts things in her mouth now.'

So, first stop, family and friends. If things are complicated or if you feel it might help anyway you could try professional help.

Professionals

You might find it useful to discuss tricky points with a psychologist who is interested in behavioural methods and is using these methods with children with learning disabilities. If you have difficulty finding someone in your area, write to the British Psychological Society at the address given in Appendix 2.

If your child is at school her teacher may be able to help and may anyway be interested to hear what you are trying to do. Other interested people – your doctor or social worker, speech- or physiotherapist, people at the Toy Library, nursery school, school, clinic, hospital – might be glad to know what you are doing and, where possible, may tailor their efforts to fit in with yours. Love makes the world go round but communication gives it a good push in the right direction.

If you feel like not only getting help for yourself but also helping others and sharing problems and victories in a big way you could think about contacting other people to form a group.

Getting a group together

If you don't know other parents of children with learning disabilities, write to MENCAP at the address given in Appendix 2 and the agency's divisional general manager may be able to put you in touch with other parents in your area.

Finally, behavioural methods have helped some parents to see their children in a new light.

'Since I have been using these methods I feel more able to control Evan and find it easier to be one jump ahead of him. Disabled he may be but he's aware of what he's doing and knows right from wrong. I think, too, that he wasn't stretched enough, I was doing too much for him. Now I expect, and get, more from him and I'm pleased, and he's pleased I'm pleased!'

'Behavioural methods show you how to sort your problems out and stop you getting too cross with the child so you can build up a better relationship between you.'

'We are such good friends now, Ann and I, we do so much more together. I find her so much more rewarding now. It just changes your whole attitude.'

Children with special disabilities

Behavioural methods can be used to help all sorts of children, not only those with disabilities. However, children with special disabilities – blindness, deafness, cerebral palsy, spina bifida, and many other forms of disability – do have special problems which may affect their learning. It is not possible in this book to go into ways of tackling all these different kinds of problems in detail, but you can get a great deal of help from the various agencies listed in Appendix 2. A number of books dealing with particular disabilities are also listed in Appendix 3.

Children with autism, and the problems they present, perhaps deserve special mention. The majority of these children have learning disabilities, and their parents, and others who work with them, may turn to a book such as this one for help. They may feel that although many of the methods described here can be used effectively with children with autism, in some cases they have to be tailored to the specific needs of these children.

Space does not allow for discussion here, but there are two books in which the methods are described, particularly as they apply to children with autism, the details of which are given in Appendix 3.

The practice problems

At the end of each chapter you will find a short section called 'Some practice problems'. These were at first intended as light relief, and you can treat them as such. Later it became clear that they might have a more useful purpose: as a way of working out methods and solutions for problems other than those you are immediately concerned with, giving you the opportunity to think about new situations and to try to be flexible and imaginative about them. So, if you like, work out your own answers to the 'practice problems', perhaps as revision.

In some of the 'practice problems' I have suggested you look at your own family situation, and only you will know the answers to these. In others, the ones which are starred, the questions are more general, and some general answers are given in Appendix 1. But remember, the 'practice problems' were originally included for a bit of fun and relaxation, so don't take them too seriously.

Part 1: Ways of Teaching

2. Observation: Watching and Counting

Observation is the cornerstone of behavioural methods. Everything we do starts with observation, and depends on observation. From our observations we decide on the problem, what we should do about it, and whether what we are doing is making a difference.

How to observe

The main reasons for wanting to make observations are: first, to get things clear – to define the 'good' or the 'bad' behaviour; secondly, to get them expressed in precise rather than vague words; thirdly, to pin them down to events or patterns of behaviour which can be counted.

Suppose a mother says, 'What *can* I do about Jill, she's really awful these days?' We would ask in what *way* Jill is awful. 'Well, she never leaves me alone, she's always following me around – and she won't do a thing I tell her to do.' Suppose we know that Jill is about 8 years old – that is, she is not a tiny child in whom this kind of behaviour would be fairly normal – we would want to know more. Is there any particular time that Jill follows her mother around? Does she do it more in the morning before school? Or in the evening? Or at weekends? Is she said to be disobedient at school? Does she follow her father or other adults too? Is she disobedient to her father? Are there any special requests that she won't obey? Or that she will – if her mother says, 'Help yourself to a biscuit', does she disobey that? Does she follow her mother (or other people) only at home? Or does she follow her in other places as well? Does it make any difference if other people are present? What does her mother do when Jill follows her

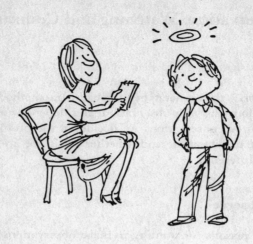

around? Or won't obey her? How does Jill react to this?

By now we should have a fairly clear idea, from the mother's description, of Jill's difficult behaviour. Ideally we would now watch Jill and her mother together for some time to see what actually happens, though you can be sure that if we were sitting around waiting to see Jill being tiresome she would behave like an angel all afternoon. (Outside observers often turn out to alter the behaviour they are there to observe, though if they stay long enough and don't chat to the person they are observing things usually go back to 'normal'.) One way or another we should be able to collect enough information to make a clear definition, with her mother, of the tiresome things Jill does.

'Following round' might be defined as Jill being close to her mother – say within about three feet of her – and not occupied with something on her own (not counting times when Jill and her mother are going somewhere or doing something together, like going shopping or for walks). 'Disobedience' might be defined as any time that Jill is asked or told to do something and she does not begin to do it within about five seconds of the request. These definitions sound quite reasonable, though we may find that as we begin to use them we have to redefine them again and again, to get them clear.

Having decided on and defined the kinds of behaviour we want to work on we are now ready to begin to count and to record how often they occur.

Recording observations

There are several reasons why we should put our observations down on paper, rather than keep them in our heads. Keeping written records will help us make the observations more carefully – it seems to matter more what we observe if the observations are going down in black and white; it makes the observations permanent, so that we can look back on what happened days or weeks ago without having to rely on memory; and, following on from this, it cuts out the arguments between different people as to when or how much of the behaviour really occurred.

Different ways of recording

Records can be kept in a number of different ways, and we can use the one which best suits us, and the problem, at the time.

1. Continuous recording

This is the 'diary' method. *The observer tries to write down everything that happens.* Since it is physically impossible to write everything down, she records some things and misses out others so of course two people observing the same child at the same time would not necessarily record the same things. It is an exhausting procedure, and is not much used in behavioural work. Nevertheless it can be a good way to make preliminary

observations of a child's behaviour, especially for someone
who does not know the child well, like a new nurse or teacher.

2. Event recording

*The observer selects one or more particular kinds of behaviour,
and records every time they occur.* For instance, we could record
how many times a child came when she was called, or used her
potty, or threw something, or took off her socks. The record
may be taken over any period of time. If the behaviour happens
only occasionally, the record may be taken over the whole day;
if frequently, it may be more convenient to record it over a
particular half hour or hour. Jill's disobedience could be recorded like this: her mother could record how often Jill did not
comply with a request from the time she got up in the morning
until she left for school, and again when she came back from
school until, say, 6 in the evening or until she was in bed.
Times can be chosen which are convenient for the person
doing the recording.

Event recording is a simple straightforward procedure and
used a good deal in practical situations.

3. Duration recording

The observer records how long a certain piece of behaviour lasts.
This is used for the kinds of behaviour that are not exactly
events, as they are not on-off affairs, like a throw or a kick, but
once started normally last for some time, like running; in this
case it may seem better to record not how often the bit of
behaviour happens but how long it lasts. For instance, we
would use duration recording to record how long a child
spends smiling or playing with a toy.

When a programme was devised to try to give Geoffrey,
who was deaf and could not speak, a happier, more enriched
life, its effect on him (that is, whether the programme had
actually resulted in his being happier) was measured by recording whether he smiled more when the programme was in place

than he did before, and duration recording was the method used for this.

Jill's mother might use this method for the 'following round' problem: she might record how much time Jill spends within three feet of her, or she might record the time Jill spends further than three feet away from her, if this were likely to be less. Again, Jill's mother could choose the times in which she would keep her records to suit herself.

A stopwatch is a help in duration recording, but not essential. Paula's mother, who was trying to teach her to keep her mouth closed to stop her constant dribbling, used to sit opposite the kitchen clock for her five-minute sessions, and record the number of seconds in the five minutes that Paula's mouth was actually closed. (Once the record showed that it had been closed for eight minutes: 'It was going so well, and all that time she was *swallowing*, I just didn't stop.')

4. *Partial interval recording*

The observer divides up the time in which she will make her observations into certain periods, or intervals – say, five minutes, ten minutes, thirty seconds, one day, or whatever she chooses. Then *she records whether or not the behaviour happened at all during that interval*. It would make no difference to the record whether the behaviour happened once or fifty times in any one interval: the record simply states that the behaviour did or did not happen.

This is a simple kind of recording which can be used instead of either event or duration recording. It also makes it easier to record more than one piece of behaviour at a time. Jill's mother could divide up the time after Jill gets back from school into quarter-hour intervals: she could then record, for each quarter hour, whether Jill had, at any time in the quarter hour, been further than three feet away from her, and whether she had obeyed any request. (Jill's mother chose to make her records this way: that is, instead of counting the bad behaviour, 'disobedience' and 'following round', she counted how often

Jill behaved well, 'obedience' and 'not following round'. She thought this would be easier – 'there'll be nothing on the charts'. She was surprised to find that she was not quite right about this, and that Jill *was* sometimes obedient and did not *always* cling to her like a limpet.) A tick would show that Jill *had* been more than three feet away, or had obeyed a request, and a cross would show the opposite. In the 'obedience' row a nought (o) would show that Jill's mother had not asked her to do anything in that interval. The record might look something like this:

	3.30–3.45	3.45–4	4–4.15	4.15–4.45	4.30–5.30				5.30–6.30			
Distance	×	×	×	√	√	×	√	×	×	×	×	×
Obedience	o	×	√	×	×	o	o	×	o	×	×	×

So for these three hours it would be clear that Jill had moved away from her mother in three of the twelve intervals, and had obeyed a request in one. We can also see a hint that Jill became more clinging and disobedient towards the end of the evening, though more records would be needed to discover whether this was a regular pattern.

The tricky part of this kind of recording is that the observer has to keep alert to the passing of time, or several intervals may go by without the behaviour being recorded. It can also require a lot of concentration, especially if the behaviour does not occur, as this means that the observer has to keep on watching like a hawk throughout the entire interval (whereas if the behaviour occurred she could record a tick and then relax for the rest of the interval).

It helps to set a kitchen timer to go off at the end of the interval, resetting it each time it goes off.

5. *Momentary time-sampling*

Here too the period under observation is divided up into intervals, but in this case the observer records whether the behaviour is happening at one moment *only*, usually at the end of the interval. So Jill's mother might record whether Jill was more than three feet away from her at the moment before 3.45, 4 o'clock and so on.

The advantage of this method over partial interval recording is that it does not require such prolonged attention on the part of the observer, and so may be more manageable. When Tess was learning not to put brushes in her mouth her parents began by using interval recording. As Tess got better and put fewer brushes in her mouth, they found interval after interval going by which needed a lot of their attention and ended with a cross for 'no behaviour seen'. While they were pleased with this it was taking up a lot of their time, so they switched to momentary time sampling instead, which left them free to get on with other things.

Once again, a kitchen timer will let you know when to make the observation.

You may have noticed that none of these methods is likely to catch every occurrence of the behaviour. You could only hope to do this if there was somebody to watch the child every minute of the day. Few of us can do that: we have other things to do with our lives. So we have to accept that we miss some instances of the behaviour and that our records are partial; nevertheless they give us a clearer idea of what is going on than if we had kept no written records and had just relied on memory.

Baselines

The most important reason for making and recording observations is to enable us to judge whether what we are doing is having the effect we want on the child's behaviour – whether she is any 'better', following our efforts, than she was before. This means that we need a record of what she was like before we started to teach her something, to compare with later records. The record of what the behaviour is like before we start trying to change it is called a *baseline*.

Sometimes people are reluctant to spend time taking a baseline, especially if the behaviour is an unpleasant or destructive one, in which case they want to start work to discourage it as quickly as possible. As a rule, though, a baseline is helpful because, with it, we can see more clearly the effect of what we are doing, whereas if we started straight in with our treatment we might not be sure what change was taking place.

Baselines can give us all sorts of useful information. In her baseline Jill's mother might have found that Jill was more likely to be difficult late in the evening, perhaps when she was tired, or when visitors came to the house; that she was more likely to obey requests made by her father than by her mother, or vice versa. One thing Jill's mother would be quite likely to find is that Jill is actually more obedient and less continuously difficult than she thought. Just counting these things often helps to put them in perspective.

There is one other benefit, one that is unusual but which I have encountered often enough that I am no longer astounded by it: sometimes simply taking a baseline resolves the problem.

In one case, some nurses at a hospital wanted to treat a boy who was banging his head. They decided to take a baseline, simply recording how often he banged his head each day. To their amazement, as they began to record the baseline, he began to bang his head less and less until he finally stopped doing it altogether. They never found out for certain what brought about this change, though they suspected that, in some strange way, the boy was affected by the fact that every time he banged, someone in the room reached for a pencil and made a mark on paper, but it did mean they did not need to embark on 'treatment'.

Graphs

When we keep records most of us will add up the figures, over the day or the week, to see how things are going and whether any change can be seen over the days or weeks. Some people like to put these figures on a chart, or graph, as this pictorial kind of record gives them a more vivid impression than they get from just looking at the figures. Timmy's mother kept records of his tantrums, using the back of an old calendar which she stuck up on the kitchen wall: each day she wrote down the day and the date, and then every time Timmy had a tantrum she put a tick under that day. As the treatment she was using began to take effect the tantrums became fewer. After a while Timmy's mother made up a chart and entered her figures on it. By now she had been keeping a record for quite some time, so to save space she added up all the figures for each week and divided them by seven, giving her an average daily figure for each week. She had taken a two-week baseline and used the treatment for six weeks, so her graph looked like this:

Tantrums

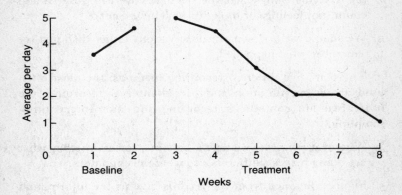

This story has rather a happy ending. The school that Timmy went to had not wanted to tackle his tantrums in the way that his mother was using (*extinction*, see page 88–92) as they did not think it would work. After she had drawn up the graph, Timmy's mother took it along to the school and showed it to the teachers. They were surprised and impressed, and were convinced by this evidence that what she was doing was after all a useful approach to the problem of Timmy's tantrums.

Keeping records can seem a tiresome chore at the time but later it can be very gratifying to look back and see how much the child has progressed. As one parent has said: 'The keeping of regular records is useful as one sometimes does not realize how quick progress has been; it also helps one to spot difficulties and areas where one should try a new approach.'*

The main points

1. In making observations we want to:
   (a) be quite clear about exactly what the child does;
   (b) describe what she does clearly, not vaguely;
   (c) describe things that she does that we can observe and count (not feelings or thoughts which we can't).

2. We should write down our observations rather than just try to remember what happened.

3. There are five different recording methods; the most often used are event, duration and partial interval recording; the other two are continuous recording and momentary time-sampling.

4. Wherever possible, we take a baseline, to see whether what we are doing makes a difference to what the child does.

5. Figures obtained from the records give us the information more vividly if presented as a graph.

* Ronald Brown, *One in Seven is Special*, NSMHC, 1974.

Some practice problems

1. Keep a record of some unimportant happening in your home: how often one child goes upstairs or into the garden; or says 'Please' or 'No' – anything you like.
Use any one of the recording methods suggested.
Do it for any length of time you like – all day or only part of each day. If you decide to use only part of a day use the same part or parts each day you make your observations.

2. Try setting your record out on a graph.

3. Reinforcement: 'You've Done It – Hurray!'

Reinforcement is a familiar word. We talk of reinforcements for an army, of reinforced concrete, of reinforcing the seat of a small boy's pants. In each case what we are talking about is strengthening something: extra troops to bolster up those already in the field, iron girders set into concrete to toughen it, extra material in that part of the pants where strength is most needed. When the word *reinforcement* is used in behavioural work it has the same meaning, but since we are now talking about behaviour, what we mean is: *reinforcement strengthens behaviour*.

Reinforcement is anything which, when it follows a piece of behaviour, results in an increase in that behaviour in the future:

Adult says: 'Sit down'	Child sits down	Adult says: 'That's lovely', and gives a kiss	Child sits down more readily next time she is asked
Behaviour		*Reinforcement*	*Result*

Everyone depends to some extent on reinforcement for their actions. If you think carefully about any aspect of your everyday life you will see that most of what you do is in the expectation of some form of reinforcement (though sometimes this may be something that will happen well into the future).

The same is true for children with learning disabilities. They too need reinforcement, especially when the things we would like them to do are not particularly interesting or enjoyable to them. We may need to plan reinforcement deliberately for the learning-disabled child because there may not be many things in her life that she enjoys so much that she is willing to work for them – that is, that are reinforcing to her; she may be less able than we are to look to the future or to wait for reinforcement; and she may be less able to get reinforcement from very small things happening around her – for instance, a slight smile on her mother's face. So it often turns out that she does not get much reinforcement at all. When this happens she may give up expecting it, and feel there is little point in making an effort to do things: she then seems to be lazy, and we say 'she won't try'.

Reinforcement is one of the keys to learning for the child with learning disabilities. When we reinforce her after her good behaviours we help her to learn. Many parents do this anyway. A child just learning to use her potty may get a delighted hug and a kiss from her mother the first time she actually performs in it; this makes it more likely that she will use her potty next time she sits on it. It does not make it certain, but, providing of course that she likes hugs and kisses, it makes it more likely than if there had been no hugs or kisses.

You will remember that reinforcement is *anything* that makes a piece of behaviour more likely to occur. We should never assume that any particular thing is a reinforcer for any particular person, though some things *are* found to be reinforcing for most people. Many children with learning disabilities are willing to make an effort if they know that this will be followed by a sweet or a biscuit, but some are not. So in every case where we want a child to learn we have to find out what *she* is so keen on that she will work for it. When we have found it, that is a reinforcer for her.

Kinds of reinforcers

There are four main kinds of reinforcers:

1. *Primary reinforcers*

These are the things that are necessary for life – food, drink, warmth, sleep. The first two are quite often used with children, the third and fourth hardly ever. Food and drink are powerful reinforcers because they are such basic needs. Primary reinforcers, naturally enough, work better when the child actually needs them – food when she is hungry, drinks when she is thirsty. However, she is unlikely ever to be so hungry or so thirsty that just any food or drink will do; we have to look around for her favourites to use them as reinforcers.

2. *Secondary or generalized reinforcers*

These are things that, although not useful in themselves to the child, become valued because they make it possible for her to get what she wants. Money is a good example of a secondary reinforcer. In itself it does nothing for us but it can be exchanged for things we want and so it has great value for us. Similarly, tokens or stars or points that the child earns can be exchanged in the same way. Secondary reinforcers are not always easy to use, especially with children with very severe disabilities, but if they can be used they have some special advantages.

Using secondary reinforcers is described more fully in chapter 4, 'Star charts and tokens'.

3. *Social reinforcers*

Praise, smiles, hugs, kisses, cuddles; anything that involves giving attention. Just a glance or a raised eyebrow can sometimes work as a reinforcer, and even crossness can be a reinforcer: if the child desperately wants attention, angry attention may be better than none at all. She may also find it very simple to get angry attention just by behaving badly.

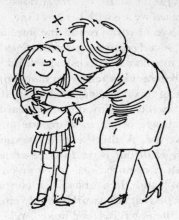

4. *Stimulating reinforcers*

There are a number of things which a child can find reinforcing which are neither primary, secondary, nor social: toys, games and activities; music; bright lights; other kinds of sights, sounds and sensations. These seem to be reinforcing because the child enjoys the stimulation, the interesting experience, she gets from them.

Finding reinforcers for the individual child

Many children enjoy and will work for food reinforcers. Sweets, of course, spring to mind, and if that is what the child likes best then they may be what we have to use. Sweets and sweet things are, however, bad for the children's teeth and liable to make them fat, so wherever possible we look for other foods that they like – cheese, crisps, fruit, sultanas, carrots. Drinks too are often reinforcing to children: orange or other juices, milk, tea, coffee – sometimes just water.

Other children love attention, praise, hugs and kisses – the social reinforcers. In many ways these are the reinforcers that most of us would prefer to use wherever possible. We can show the child how pleased we are with her any time, whereas it is more complicated to have to carry round the special toys or bits of apple. Moreover, social reinforcers are the ones we get in normal everyday life for most small successes; a child who responds to them is that much nearer her fellow human beings than one who does not. Because of this it is always to be hoped that a child who is not interested in social reinforcers can learn to enjoy them, so they should always be given alongside any other kind of reinforcer that we use. A child who is not specially interested in praise from an adult but is mad on ice-cream should, when she has done what is required of her, be given a hug and told, 'That's splendid!', and then given a spoonful of ice-cream. Eventually we hope that the two kinds of reinforcement – the social and the edible – will become linked in her mind, she will come to enjoy the praise and the hug, and both will become reinforcing to her.

Some children show little response to praise and attention, and may not be particularly interested in food. In this situation we have to explore other things that may be reinforcing, and may have to be imaginative and ingenious about it. Here are a few things that have been found reinforcing for some children:

1. music – records, tapes, singing;
2. clapping;
3. stroking, tickling, patting;
4. 'frolicking' – being bounced or jumped;
5. bright lights – a torch to switch on;
6. hand cream rubbed on to the child's hand;
7. sucking an ice cube;
8. an electric toothbrush.

Sometimes reinforcers are found which are very idiosyncratic indeed. One boy had 'a passion for hot jam-filled pancakes'.* This caused some problems of handling and delivery – how to

* M. C. Jones, *Behaviour Problems in Handicapped Children*, London, Souvenir Press, 1983, p. 158.

keep the pancakes hot throughout a teaching session? How to give them in small enough bits? What about all the washing-up afterwards? Fortunately the boy could manage tokens, which he earned in the teaching sessions and exchanged later, at lunchtime, for the pancakes.

In another case, a mother, asked what would be good reinforcers for her severely disabled 14-year-old daughter, said, 'Oh, I know exactly. Gloves and stockings'. But what this meant was, not, as you may have thought, gifts of gloves and stockings but the sensation of having gloves pulled over her hands and of stockings pulled on over her legs. These very unusual reinforcers may be of crucial importance for some children, so we have to be prepared to search for them.

Where it is very difficult to think of anything that the child is really keen on we may make use of the *Premack Principle* (David Premack is an American psychologist who first defined the principle). According to this any activity that the child does frequently when left to herself may be used as a reinforcer. For instance, if a child spends much of her time running around, or rocking, then we may allow her to run or rock *only* when she has performed some task that we want her to do. Probably most of us would not ordinarily think of these things, running, or rocking or, in the case of Timmy, twiddling a plastic cup on his thumb (see pages 172–3) as particularly reinforcing, and would not think of using them as reinforcers. But if a particular child demonstrates a 'preferred activity' – that is, she behaves in a particular way whenever she can – then this is a hint that her behaviour could be used to reinforce her learning of other things. So if we want the running-about child to learn to sit still she may learn to do so if she is only allowed to run when she has sat still for a short time. It sounds mad, but it can work.

You will see that selecting a good reinforcer for a child is a matter of very careful observation of what she enjoys most and of what she likes best to do. Parents are often very good at this, as they know the child so well, and may notice things about her that other people miss.

It is important to remember that a reinforcer, which increases the behaviour it follows, will have this sort of effect on any kind of behaviour, good or bad. No one sets out deliberately to make a child do bad things more often, but we may, in fact, do so without realizing it. For example, a child who enjoys adult attention may find that a certain way to get attention is to throw ornaments through the window, or attack her baby brother – people rush to her side, they hold her, look earnestly at her, make gestures and talk to her. For some time following her action she can rely on being the centre of attention. Next time she feels in need of attention, wham goes another flower vase.

Of course, nobody would deliberately increase the number of times a child did these things: but if she is reinforced by attention, and if her bad behaviour is followed by attention, this behaviour may continue or become more frequent. Once we have identified the reinforcers for a child we should try to make sure they follow her good behaviours, and not her bad ones. (See also chapter 7, pages 88–9.)

Positive reinforcement and negative reinforcement

Up till now I have been talking about positive reinforcement. This is by far the most important kind of reinforcement, used to increase skills and add to the fun the child has. However, people quite often talk about 'negative reinforcement', implying that this is what to use when the child behaves badly, so perhaps I should explain the meaning of the term.

At the beginning of this chapter we said that *reinforcement strengthens behaviour*. This is true of both positive reinforcement and negative reinforcement, but they do it in different ways: positive reinforcement works by following a piece of behaviour by *giving something good*; negative reinforcement works by following a piece of behaviour by *taking away something bad*. So negative reinforcement is another way of *increasing* behaviour, and is not a way to stop behaviours happening.

Negative reinforcement is hardly ever used deliberately with children, though adults quite often find it working on them. Suppose Rupert hears the chimes of the ice-cream van and runs to his mother: 'Mum, can I have a lolly?' His mother doesn't think he should have one and says so. 'Oh, go on, Mum, let me have a lolly, I *do* want one. *Everybody's* out there, I'm the *only* one in the street who isn't getting a lolly! Go on, Mum, I haven't had one for *ages*. It's only 35p. I'll be *ever* so good if you let me. *Go* on, Mum.' And so on and on. At last his mother gives him the 35p. Rupert runs off, the pestering stops and his mother thinks, 'Well it was worth letting him have the money for the lolly, it will keep him quiet for a bit.' Her giving in is negatively reinforced, through the relief it brings her from the pestering. She may be more likely to hand over the lolly money more readily next time. (Unless, of course, she tumbles to the fact that at the same time Rupert is being positively reinforced for pestering and is likely to pester more. Once she realizes that she may decide to take a firm stand.)

Negative reinforcement can work on adults, as it did on Rupert's mother. Because the effect is to relieve the adult from some unpleasant or stressful situation, adults may go along with it, and this may be why they go on using methods that are really not worthwhile. The mother who said that smacking did not change the child's behaviour was nevertheless still smacking her daughter, because 'it stops her at the time' (see page 97). Stopping her *at the time* made the mother feel better, but it was not the best way of dealing with the behaviour. We need to be aware of the effects that negative reinforcement may have on us, and try to make sure they do not lead us up the garden path.

How to give reinforcement

1. Reinforcement should be given when the child does what we want her to and not, as far as possible, at other times; this

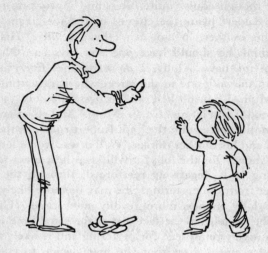

helps to keep her interested in the reinforcer. Of course, I don't mean that if attention is the reinforcer we never attend to the child unless, say, she puts the yellow brick in the yellow box. That would be absurd. Of course she receives attention in the ordinary way during the course of the day. But in the ten minutes or so that are set aside to teach her she gets our warmest praise, our most enthusiastic hugs and kisses, for those times when she does the thing we want her to learn. So, during most of the ten minutes we remain our calm friendly selves, but when the yellow brick goes in the yellow box we go really wild.

Where the reinforcer is something other than attention it may help if we see that the child does not get too much of it at other times. Jay's mother, after discussing a programme that was having only moderate success, said thoughtfully, 'I think perhaps she's getting too many biscuits and sweets at other times. If I cut those down a bit she may be more excited about them when we do our sessions.'

2. Reinforcement should be given *immediately* after the good

behaviour. Even quite a short delay (five seconds) between the behaviour taking place and the reinforcer being given can slow down learning. This means that we need to have the reinforcer ready to hand – actually in our fingers – to give as soon as the child has done what we want.

3. Reinforcement should be given *clearly*. This applies particularly to social reinforcement: praise should be enthusiastic, smiles delighted, hugs and kisses warm. Besides being exciting and enjoyable to the child (most children anyway) this also lets her know without any doubt that she has done the right thing (see also page 78).

I said just now that warm, lively attention is enjoyable for the child. There are exceptions. Some children do not like frenetic things going on around them, even if they are at the centre. For some children (particularly, but not only, some children with autism) this can be a turn-off, so that they shrink away from it. In this case our enthusiasm would not be a reinforcer, and might even weaken the behaviour we are trying to strengthen. Once again it is a matter of careful observation of the individual child and of finding the reinforcers that will work for her.

Giving reinforcement for periods of time

I have talked about reinforcing 'a piece of behaviour', and often this is what we do, especially when the child is learning some task or skill. But there are occasions when it is more appropriate to give the reinforcement after a period of time. For example, if the child is learning to stay on a chair, or to occupy herself with a toy, we would reinforce her after, say, each five or ten seconds during which she had remained on the chair or played with the toy. Later, as she got better at what she was doing, we could lengthen the times, a little at first, and then gradually more and more. Later still we might reinforce her, sometimes after quite a short interval, sometimes after a longer one – the 'dodging around' technique, which is described below.

This way of giving reinforcement, giving it after intervals in which the good behaviour has been shown, is especially valuable when we come to tackling problem behaviours, when one of the most useful things we can do is to reinforce intervals in which the problem behaviour has *not* occurred (see page 87).

How often to give the reinforcement

When a child is learning something new we reinforce her *consistently*, every time she does it. Later, when she becomes more skilful, and succeeds with the task quite often, it is better to give the reinforcement only every now and again. So for building up a new kind of behaviour we reinforce her consistently; for keeping the behaviour going once she has begun to gets the hang of it we reinforce her intermittently, every now and again. The reason for this move is, first, that as the child gets more skilful she can produce the behaviour more easily and quickly; if every piece of behaviour were reinforced she might get too much and get tired of it. Secondly, the every-now-and-again kind of reinforcement seems better at keeping the behaviour going. This may be because of its unpredictability: if you have ever played on a fruit machine, you may have put in another coin because even though you did not win last time you might the next; and so you went on trying.

The fruit machine analogy also gives us a guide to how the every-now-and-again reinforcement should be paced. If we play on the machine for too long and it does not give us anything at all, we are likely to give up in disgust and turn away. So we do not let too long a time go by before we give the reinforcement. This is especially important at first. When we first decide that it is time to stop giving the reinforcement for every piece of behaviour, we should not leave long gaps between reinforcers; indeed at this early stage it is a good idea occasionally to give reinforcement straight after a piece of the behaviour (like we did when we were using consistent reinforcement, only then we did this every time). So Ben, who was learning to put the table knives away in the knife drawer and was getting rather good at it, might get his reinforcement after he put away the first knife, then after the fourth then after the sixth, then after the seventh, and the eighth, then after the twelfth. At the end of this he has put away a dozen knives and has had reinforcement six times. However, these times were dodged around, so he was never quite sure when the reinforcement would come, but because it came quite often he did not lose heart but was willing to go on working for it. Later, as Ben becomes even more adept at the task, it should be possible to space out the reinforcers further until he may only need it when all the knives have been put away, or may not need it at all. (See 'How to end a token programme', pages 53–5.)

The main points

1. Reinforcement is anything which, when it follows immediately on a piece of behaviour, makes it more likely that the piece of behaviour will occur again.

2. Reinforcers may be:
   (*a*) primary – things to eat or drink;
   (*b*) secondary – stars, tokens, money, which can be exchanged for whatever the person wants;
   (*c*) social – attention, praise, smiles, hugs, kisses, cuddles;
   (*d*) stimulating – toys, games, activities, sights, sounds and sensations.

3. Positive reinforcement works by following the behaviour by giving something good: negative reinforcement by taking away something bad. Both increase behaviour.

4. The reinforcement we use in behavioural work is almost always *positive*.

5. We look for whatever the child is *really* fond of, fond enough to be willing to work for it, to use as a reinforcer for her.

6. The *Premack Principle* means using as a reinforcer anything that the child does frequently when left to herself – a
preferred activity.

7. Reinforcement should be given only for the kinds of behaviour we want the child to show.

8. Reinforcement should be given:
   (*a*) when the child shows the good behaviour;
   (*b*) immediately she shows the behaviour; and
   (*c*) clearly – especially the social reinforcers.

9. When the child is learning something new it is best to give
the reinforcement consistently, every time it is shown.

10. To keep the behaviour going it is better to give the reinforcement only every now and again.

11. When we start giving the reinforcement every now and
again it is important to give it still quite often. Later the
intervals between reinforcers can be increased.

Some practice problems

1. List some things that you think may be reinforcing for
your child.

2. List some things you think would be reinforcing for you.
Which of the four headings (primary, secondary, social, stimulating) would each of these come under?

3. Can you think of any time when, without meaning to, you
reinforced one of your child's bad behaviours?

*4. Can you think of some everyday activity of yours that does
not bring you much reinforcement from other people (i.e. the

* 'Practice problems' marked with an asterisk throughout the book are more
general and have some general answers. These are given in Appendix 1, pages
207–21, at the back of the book.

reinforcement normally comes only from your own feeling of having done it well)? How much difference would it make if somebody reinforced you for this every time you did it? Or just now and again?

*5. *Scene*: A hotel lounge. A guest is lurking in the background (writing this book actually). Enter a mother and father and pretty little girl of about three.

    Child: 'Mummy, I've got a pain.'

    Mother: 'Where does it hurt?'

    Child: (indicates an improbable area near her armpit)

    Father: 'Never mind, have a sweetie.' (Addressing the guest) 'We find that soon cures it.'

    Guest: (thinks)

Who here is being negatively reinforced? And who positively? What do you think will be the outcome? Would you (if asked) suggest that the parents do anything differently?

4. Star Charts and Tokens

Stars and tokens are one kind of reinforcer. Like points and counters, they are *secondary* reinforcers: when the child does what we want her to do she is given a star or a token which she can later exchange for something she wants.

Stars and tokens work in much the same way that money does. In itself money is of little use to us – we can't eat a coin or drink a five pound note. We all know, however, that if we have money we can use it to exchange for food or drink or whatever else we want, so in our society money is valued. In the same way when the child finds that if she gets a star now she will be able to exchange it later for something she wants, she will come to value the stars: they become reinforcing to her. When she is given a star following something she does, she is more likely to do that thing again.

Many people may not want to use stars or tokens – some will have no need of them, or of the other suggestions in this book, others may feel they do not want to use this method – and they should not concern themselves with this chapter. But for some children, and their parents, it offers another and often highly enjoyable kind of help.

Why we use stars or tokens

Stars or tokens are especially useful with older or rather brighter children. For these children many of the reinforcers discussed earlier (chapter 3) are of little interest: these children are not thrilled by bites of food, sips of drink or snatches of music. What they are interested in is, perhaps, something more substantial: pop CDs, a transistor radio, new clothes, extra swimming sessions or meals in a restaurant. If the child is really keen on these things we want to be able to make use of them as reinforcers, but because they are large and expensive things, or because they may be difficult to give quickly we cannot use them in the same way as pieces of cheese or crisps: we cannot give a child a transistor radio each time she tidies her bedroom, or take her swimming each time she is helpful in the house. Instead the child can work towards her chosen reinforcer, earning stars (or tokens or points or whatever) for each piece of good behaviour, until at last she has enough to exchange for the reinforcer.

Besides helping the child to learn, stars may also help to make life pleasanter all round. Parents who have found themselves driven to nagging can let the stars take over; the nagging stops; the child has a straightforward choice between doing what she is asked and getting a star for it or not doing the task and forgoing the star. Without the nagging, life becomes more peaceful. For the parents, too, giving the star is a useful reminder to give social reinforcement ('Here's your star, Gary. Well done, you did do that nicely!') so the child benefits in both ways. Of course the parents could have given the praise all along without waiting for the star. But parents are human, too; in everyday life opportunities seem to slip by, while having a programme to follow may make it more likely that the opportunities will be taken. Many parents who have tried using stars have been surprised and delighted at the change in the child, at how much more eager and willing she is to cooperate pleasantly when the reinforcement she wants actually comes her way.

Another reason for using stars or tokens can be to save the interruption that using ordinary reinforcers entails. Colin, who was 18 years old, attended his local day centre and sat there, rocking, day after day. It seemed impossible to get him to participate in the centre's activities. At last it was discovered that he was very fond of orange juice, and using sips of this as a reinforcer he started to take part in the activities. As he began to participate more he moved on to receiving tokens, which he exchanged at the end of the session for a glass of orange juice. So he did not have to stop what he was doing to take a sip and he had a really satisfying drink at the end. Interestingly, Colin, who had been reluctant at first to take part in the activities, came to enjoy them so much that within two or three weeks he no longer needed the tokens or the orange juice: the activities themselves became reinforcing and he would do other useful things, like learning to wash his hands, if afterwards he could go back to the activities. The reinforcers had opened up new experiences for him and allowed him to find out how much he enjoyed them.

Setting up a programme

There are four main steps in setting up this kind of programme. We have to decide on:
1. The kind of behaviour we want to change.
2. How many stars will be given for the things the child does.
3. The exchange reinforcers – what she can get for her stars.
4. How many stars are to be given in exchange for the reinforcer.

1. *Deciding what behaviour we want to change*

We can use stars just like other reinforcers, either to encourage or to discourage something the child does: either to increase the number of times she behaves well, for instance by being friendly to her brother or getting dressed in the morning; or to decrease the number of times she behaves badly, perhaps grinding her teeth or swearing. If we want to increase a good behaviour we have to make as careful a definition of it as we can and follow the good behaviour with a star. If we want the child to stop doing something we may use DRO – *Differential Reinforcement of Other kinds of behaviour* (see pages 86–8). Here, instead of defining the bad behaviour that we want to get rid of, we focus on others that we want to encourage to take the place of the bad behaviour. In many cases these 'Other' kinds of behaviour that we want to increase will be the opposite of the bad behaviours that we want to decrease: we would reinforce the child for *not* grinding her teeth or for *not* swearing. For example, Ann was very disobedient and disobliging, and her mother wanted to help her get over this. She set up a programme in which Ann was given a star to stick on a chart every time she was obedient – that is, every time she began to do what she was asked within five seconds of her mother asking it. Dino, who made a great deal of trouble in class, was given a token for every half hour in the classroom in which he had not caused trouble. ('Not causing trouble' had to be rather carefully defined: not leaving his seat without permission, not interfering with other children, not disobeying a teacher, not grumbling or whining.)

2. *How many tokens to give*

At the beginning of a programme, this is quite easy: a star is given for every good piece of behaviour, or at regular intervals of good behaviour. It gets more complicated when we want to ask the child to do more for her stars. This is discussed under 'Adapting the programme', page 48.

3. *Deciding on the exchange reinforcers*

One of the advantages of these programmes is that we can use all sorts of reinforcers and be as imaginative as we like. I have already suggested using quite large reinforcers (transistor radio, new clothes, etc.). Parents quite often do something of the sort anyway: promise, for example, a bicycle if the child will do this or that over a period of time – pass an exam, be good until Christmas. But unless the child is very strong-willed this sort of promise often does not lead to a consistent change in her behaviour, because the reinforcer is so far away from what she is doing here and now. By giving a star for each of the individual things she does we can bring the whole idea of the reinforcement nearer, making it more real to her.

Privileges of one sort or another can be used as reinforcers: a special visit to the cinema or other treat. Sometimes, however, it's very difficult to find extra things that a child likes enough and that we can afford and we may then have to use everyday things that she is fond of which might ordinarily be regarded as hers by right.

If the child herself asks for help, we may be able to agree with her on the use of her normal rights as reinforcers – my son readily agreed that the reinforcer for his programme should be his pocket-money. If we have to use these normal 'rights' or privileges in this way, we make sure that the child can obtain the privilege quite easily, especially at first, so that she doesn't lose out.

All sorts of things may be used as reinforcers for children for whom 'extras' cannot be found; anything that the child is interested in or enjoys. Sue, who was expected to mix with the other children at her school in the normal way, very much liked to be able to get away from them and to spend time in her bedroom by herself. This was not usually allowed, as school rules said that bedrooms were out of bounds during the day but she was able to use her tokens to 'buy' time to spend in her bedroom. Rachel, on the other hand, used hers to get the chance to watch her favourite TV programme. Other children may like to earn outings, visits to the zoo, the chance to go swimming, time to spend with a favourite person, staying up later in the evening. The important thing, as with all reinforcers, is that it should be something that the child is really keen on and willing to work for. In Ann's case, for example, the psychologist working with her mother at first suggested using Ann's pocket-money, with a little extra added, and giving her one penny of her pocket-money in exchange for every four stars. At first this worked well, but one morning her mother found that Ann had ripped all her stars off her chart.

Sometimes a child will spoil her star chart in a fit of temper, wanting to show she doesn't care about it. If we think this may not be true we carry on for a while, substituting a new chart onto which any surviving stars can be re-stuck, and see whether she continues to tear up the charts or whether she really enjoys getting the stars and exchanging them for what she wants. On the other hand, the chart-spoiling may be an indication that the stars are not reinforcing for the child because the exchange items are of little interest to her. This is what happened with Ann. Her mother realized that the pennies Ann was earning in exchange for stars were simply not sufficiently reinforcing. She also knew that Ann very much wanted a particular pop CD, so this was substituted as the exchange reinforcer. As it was an expensive one she told Ann that she would have to get sixty stars in order to earn the CD, and although this took longer, it was a much more effective exchange reinforcer, and Ann went to work with a will. Not only did she obey with alacrity almost every request made of her but her mother was bombarded with offers of help on every possible occasion. Although at this point Ann was being obliging in order to get what she wanted, it was very pleasant for her mother, who in her turn responded more warmly to Ann, and the whole relationship became a happier one.

4. *Exchange rates*

There is no set way of doing this; it is a matter of trial and error. Each child, her problem, the rate at which she can earn the stars, and the exchange reinforcer that works for her, is different. We have to make an intelligent guess at a reasonable exchange rate, and then be prepared to change it if we get it wrong.

One general point is that the exchange reinforcer should be sufficiently within the child's reach: she should expect to get it with lively anticipation. To a large extent this depends on her ability to measure time, especially future time, and children vary in this. Even children with very severe disabilities can wait for half an hour or so to exchange their stars: others can wait for half a day, exchanging their stars at mid-day and again in the evening: others again can wait for a whole day, or two days, or a week, or, as in Ann's case, for several weeks. A longer wait will tend, naturally enough, to go with better (i.e. more expensive) exchange reinforcers: Lynn exchanges her stars once a day for an apple or a bar of chocolate while Philip exchanged his every four days for a small toy (see page 87). However we arrange things, we should make sure that the child continues to be keenly aware that she is, in what for her is the foreseeable future, going to get the reinforcer.

Adapting the programme

At some time in the programme we may want to make changes, either because we have not got it quite right in the first place, or because the child makes progress and we want to move things along a bit. Whichever it is, we may do one of two things: either change the rate of reinforcement (give more, or fewer, stars for the same piece of behaviour); or alter the exchange rate of stars for exchange reinforcers (make the 'price' of the exchange reinforcers higher or lower).

Making it a little easier to get reinforcement

Changes in which the child is given more stars, or is charged fewer, are usually made because it becomes apparent that we have set our sights too high. Either by giving the child too few for what she does or by expecting her to give too many in exchange (or perhaps by both) we have made it too difficult for her to get the reinforcement, with the ensuing danger that she will despair of ever being able to get it and give up trying to earn the stars. In this case we either increase the number of stars she gets or reduce the number she has to give for her reinforcers. If she has more she will be better able to 'buy' the reinforcers: or if the price of the reinforcers is lower she will have a better chance of being able to afford them. In either case the reinforcers become within her reach, and the stars are seen as leading directly to the reinforcers. The stars themselves then become reinforcing and the child will make an effort for them.

Making it a little harder to get reinforcement

The situation is rather different when the child makes good progress with her programme, begins to get plenty of stars and is often able to exchange them for the reinforcers. Not that we regret this state of affairs: it is precisely what was hoped for. It shows that the task we have set her is possible for her and that by doing it she is able to get the reinforcement. The question arises, though, of whether, if she is able to get the reinforcement so easily, she may not be doing as much as she could; alternatively she may get too much of the reinforcer too quickly and get tired of it (satiated). So we may feel that it would be better if she had to put out a bit more effort, or if the reinforcers were spaced out a little more.

The way we do this is either to decrease slightly the number of stars given for a particular piece of behaviour (so that the child has to do more to get the same number of stars): or to require slightly more stars for the reinforcer. In theory it makes little difference which of these methods we choose, but in practice it often seems easier, and less likely to cause trouble, to require more stars in exchange for the reinforcers.

How to change the programme

If the programme is for a child who can count sufficiently well we can simply tell her that she needs more stars for the reinforcer. If the child is not very good at counting but is earning stars which are put on a chart it is probably best to complete one chart and then the new one can be made a bit bigger, with extra spaces for stars; the new chart, like the old one, has to be filled up before it can be exchanged, but now it carries more stars before the goal is reached.

Again we have to be careful when adjusting the programmes that the reinforcement is not put too far out of the child's reach. The aim should always be that the child should receive adequate, even plentiful, reinforcement. After all, that is what is going to make her willing to do the things we want her to do. If we can achieve that everyone will be happy: the child getting plenty of fun and enjoyment and behaving pleasantly, cooperatively, helpfully. If the programme is adjusted because the number of stars that she is able to get has steadily increased, and consequently the amount of reinforcers that she can obtain, then the number she has to give for the reinforcer should be adjusted to that point where she gets less reinforcement than at present, but at least as much as she got at the beginning of the programme. We should not price her out of the market. In the same way, if we increase the number of stars she has to give for the reinforcer because we think she may be getting reinforcement so easily that she loses interest in it, then we should reduce the amount of reinforcement she is able to get but not by so much as to make it impossible for her to get it.

Another way of painlessly scaling up the number of stars the child has to get in order to get her reinforcer is to use new exchange reinforcers. This may be a good idea in any case in order to keep up her interest in her reinforcers. If a new reinforcer is brought into the system then the number of stars needed to get it can be made rather higher than the comparable number for the reinforcers she was getting before. For example, Ann's first exchange reinforcer was a CD, for which she had to get sixty stars. Later, when she had become very friendly and cooperative and was getting stars by the dozen, she wanted to work for a pair of pretty knickers. Although these were much cheaper to buy than the CD she was told she would need to get eighty stars for them. Compared with the CD they took a lot of stars but because Ann now gained stars quickly through her cooperative behaviour, she was able to 'buy' the knickers in about the same time that it took her to get the CD.

Fining

One of the advantages sometimes seen in star and token programmes is that they allow for stars or tokens to be taken away
in the case of bad behaviour and they have been used in this
way. Although, on the surface, these systems may be attractive
and seem to have the capacity to attack problem behaviours
directly, in reality they often break down. I have to say I have
not been very successful using fining systems for children
with learning disabilities. I do not now use them, in fact I have
not used them for years. Since I have found the programmes
much more effective when the stars or tokens were given for
good kinds of behaviour than when they were taken away for
bad ones I will not discuss fining further.

Cheating on the programme

I am talking here about cheating by adults.

Charlie's parents had asked for help with getting Charlie to
dress himself. He was slow, dreamy, and, as his parents said,
'lazy'. It would take them an hour and a half each morning to
nag him into putting on some of his clothes and eventually his
mother would dress him in the rest of them in order to have
him ready to go to school. Charlie had no actual difficulty with
managing his clothes – he was quite able to put them on and
do them up himself – so a token programme was set up by
which Charlie would be given a token for each garment that he
put on himself within a twenty-minute dressing time. Each
token was exchangeable for a little sweet which Charlie could
take with him to school.

When the psychologist went along at the end of the week to
see how things were going she found that the programme was
no longer in operation. She asked, 'Why not? Had it not
worked?'

'I'll tell you why not,' said Charlie's father. 'He was having
us on. He could do it perfectly well all the time. He came

downstairs with all his clothes on that first morning and he's done it every morning since. Today I said, "That's enough, my boy. I'm not having any more of this." All those sweets! He just couldn't be bothered, that was all there was to it. I've told him from now on he can dress himself like anybody else, to help his mother, not because he's bribed to.' When the psychologist visited the following week Charlie was once again being slow and awkward about his dressing. His father thought the whole episode proved his point – that Charlie was simply lazy.

When we set up a token programme with a child, as was done for Charlie, it is in the nature of a contract with her: the child will perform certain actions, we undertake in return to provide exchangeable tokens. The contract is drawn up on the basis that the child will be able to get a certain minimum number of tokens in order to get the exchange reinforcers. We recognize that the reason for the child's future willingness to work for the tokens – that is, to produce the behaviour that we want – is that she will, by means of the tokens, be able to obtain the exchange reinforcers. So it is essential that we should not duck out of the contract when we find that the child is successfully earning the tokens and getting the reinforcers. If we do so, not only will we have been guilty of not honouring the contract, but the child may feel, more strongly than before, the hopelessness of ever getting reinforcement.

When adults 'cheat' like this it is not as a rule because they are miserly, or that they consciously grudge the child reinforcement. The reasons are more subtle. What Charlie's father felt was typical of many in his position: that he had been conned into setting up the programme and providing the reinforcement, that Charlie was fully capable of doing what was required of him and that therefore he ought to be doing this for no reward at all but just because it was his duty as a member of the family.

Of course it is true that most children dress themselves each morning as a matter of routine and for no other reason but to allow themselves to get on with the business of the day. Let us look a little more closely at this. The child who dresses herself in order to get on with the day's business looks forward, when she is dressed, to all manner of things – an enjoyable breakfast, her comic coming with the newspapers, friends to see at school. Charlie, on the other hand, besides not being very good at looking forward, had rather little in his day to look forward to. His one real pleasure, which he could be sure he would always get, was the prolonged attention that his mother gave him over getting dressed.

What we see here is, first, that even children who apparently perform actions such as dressing with no thought of 'reward' actually do experience reinforcement for it; second, that Charlie was getting no such reinforcement; third, that when reinforcement was provided he dressed himself very well. The difference was that for Charlie the reinforcement had to be deliberately decided on and given if he was to achieve the same as other children.

So, when a programme quickly results in a child successfully performing the kind of behaviour we want of her we should not assume that she could 'do it all the time', that the programme is redundant, and that if we put a stop to it she will automatically continue to do what we want. Instead we should realize that we have found the key to this kind of behaviour for the child, and rejoice in her success: it is also ours.

How to end a token programme

A few children may need to go on getting and exchanging stars or tokens for a long time if they are to go on doing the things that we want them to, but for most the programmes need not last for ever.

Sometimes they just fade away: the child continues doing the things we want without apparently needing tokens or reinforcers. This happened with Philip (page 87) who seemed just to lose interest in his stars and the toys for which he used to exchange them, but continued sleeping through the night in his own bed. Where this happens, however, it is 'the effect of good luck, not to be reckoned on'.

In other cases the stars can be faded out because other reinforcers take over. In some of the happiest instances social reinforcers become effective, and the child continues her good behaviour because of the attention and appreciation her efforts receive. Or the activity itself may become reinforcing – she finds she likes having a tidy bedroom, or enjoys reading for its own sake – so the stars become unnecessary.

In other cases the good behaviour becomes part of the child's everyday life, and she does it as a matter of habit, but continues to need the extra pleasures she had been getting from her reinforcers. Here there is usually little difficulty in finding another skill or activity for which she can get her stars – the world is full of things for her to learn. Ann's mother went on, when disobedience and swearing were no longer a problem, to teach Ann simple cooking, knitting and household tasks, and Ann enjoyed getting stars for mastering these new tasks.

In other cases, again, we may need to stretch out the reinforcers, giving them more and more infrequently until we are giving them only very occasionally, but not doing away with them altogether. It may then be possible to stop giving the stars and give only the reinforcer in this way. Had Philip needed more help his mother might sometimes have said to him what a splendid boy he was to sleep all night in his own bed, how pleased and proud of him she and his father were; while on a very few occasions she might have added that a boy who was able to do this was so grown-up that he could probably use a few pence more in pocket-money (or something).

One last way of ending the stars or tokens is to say to the child that she has made such good progress that it seems that she no longer needs them: that the exchange reinforcers which she has been earning will now be freely available – so long as the good behaviour continues satisfactorily. If it falls off too much then we may have to set up the programme again. For example, once her temper tantrums had nearly disappeared Mandy was allowed her special biscuits every day for tea: at one time she went through a bad patch, so for a short time she had again to earn tokens and exchange them for the biscuits; the tantrums once more decreased, and after this tokens were again discontinued and have not been heard of since, and Mandy will have the biscuits every day for tea as long as she wants them.

The main points

1. Stars, tokens, points (money) are all generalized reinforcers.

2. Although not reinforcing in themselves, they can become so by being associated with other reinforcers – the exchange reinforcers.

3. Stars or tokens can be earned for good behaviour and later exchanged for the reinforcers.

4. They are especially useful for older children who are interested in larger reinforcers, or for those reinforcers that cannot be given immediately following a good behaviour.

5. In setting up a programme we have to decide on:
   (a) the good and bad behaviours and define them;
   (b) the rate of reinforcement;
   (c) the exchange reinforcer(s); and
   (d) the exchange rate of stars or tokens for reinforcers: making sure that the child has a good chance of being able to get the reinforcers.

6. We may need to adjust the programme because the child is getting either too little reinforcement or too much.

7. We can adjust the programme by changing the number of stars the child is given, or the number that she has to give for her reinforcer.

8. We should not 'cheat' by refusing to give the child reinforcement when she begins to earn it successfully.

9. The programmes can fade out:
    (a) when other reinforcers take over;
    (b) when the activity itself becomes reinforcing;
    (c) by moving the child on to learning and being reinforced for new skills;
    (d) by stretching the rate of reinforcement until the reinforcement is infrequently but still occasionally given; and
    (e) by making the reinforcement freely available to the child so long as the good behaviour continues.

Some practice problems

1. Can you think of something that anyone in your family does that you might want and be able to change using a star or token programme?

2. Which of these would be a good exchange reinforcer for you:
    (a) breakfast in bed on Sunday?
    (b) a plane ticket to Majorca?
    (c) a day off once a month?
    (d) one meal a week cooked by somebody else?
    (e) a ticket for a theatre/ballet/stock car racing/Test match/Celtic v. Rangers (or equivalent)?

Choose any two – or any two others you like. Which of your tiresome kinds of behaviour would you be prepared to modify in order to earn them?

*3. A child constantly mislays her tokens. What would you do?

*4. If you were running a programme on a desert island what would you use for tokens?

*5. People sometimes run token programmes on themselves to

help them lose weight. These programmes are often unsuccessful. Why do you think that is?

*6. Charlie's programme laid down that he would get a token for each item of clothing that he put on by himself — vest, pants, two socks, shirt, sweater and trousers; seven tokens, each one to be exchanged for a sweet. On the first morning he earned all the tokens and got all the sweets. Suppose you were Charlie's parent, and you felt he was earning the sweets too easily, what would you do?

5. Teaching by Guiding

If a child knows how to do something but is not keen on doing it, we can encourage her to do it more often by reinforcing her every time she does. However, if we want the child to learn a new activity that she has never done before, reinforcement alone is not enough – there is nothing there yet to reinforce. We need different methods to teach new skills. This chapter and the next are concerned with these methods.

What to teach and how to teach it

When we set out to teach a child something new it is important to be as sure as possible that what we are aiming to teach is something that she is capable of doing; that it is not physically impossible, or very difficult, for her. No one would try to

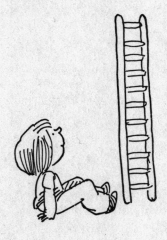

teach a child who only feeds from a bottle to feed herself with a knife and fork, or one who cannot talk to speak in sentences. A good general guideline is to teach the child something that is only just beyond her – the next step up the ladder. Also we need to make sure that the next step is a *really* small one (see page 66). This applies especially at the beginning of the teaching, because, if we hit a difficult patch, it is always worth trying the effect of putting in extra small steps in place of a bigger one (an example of this in teaching dressing is given on page 112).

The order in which most children learn things can often give an idea of what this next logical step would be. Sometimes, though, it is quite hard to know whether a skill is the right one for this child to learn at this time. Derek, who did not talk, had also not been able to learn sign language (see page 84). His teacher was uncertain whether this meant that neither speech nor sign language was a suitable communication system for him, or whether he was at that time not capable of communicating in any systematic way. She decided to go for the first possibility, that he was capable of communicating but that the two previous methods had not been suitable for him. She tried a third method, a picture language, and he picked this up quite quickly. The golden rule is: if in doubt, try it out – systematically and keeping careful records. You will soon see whether you are trying to teach something that is too hard for the child and will be able to try something else that may be better.

In this chapter I shall be discussing four main teaching methods: shaping; prompting and fading of prompts; breaking down the activity; and backward chaining; and we will also look at those useful adjuncts to teaching, structural prompts.

Shaping

Shaping means teaching the child a skill by, at first, reinforcing her for doing something that is not precisely what we want but which comes gradually closer and closer to it. Suppose we want to teach 5-year-old Kevin to use, and first of all to hold, a spoon, and we decide to do this by shaping (there are other methods we could choose which we will come to in a minute). Our baseline observations show that Kevin never holds a spoon when he is asked to, but clearly he is not deliberately being uncooperative – he just does not understand what we are saying. We cannot reinforce him for holding a spoon – he never does. He does, however, sit on a chair at the table and sometimes puts his hand on the table. So that is where we begin. We decide that when we say, 'Kevin, hold your spoon', if he puts his hand on the table he will be reinforced. In time he does this quite regularly, though his hand may be anywhere, either just in front of him or with his arm stretched along the table. We then decide that he will only be reinforced if, when he is told, 'Hold the spoon', his hand is within twelve inches of the spoon. When this becomes quite frequent he is reinforced if his hand is within nine inches of the spoon, then six inches. And so on. Gradually the criteria for reinforcement are made more and more precise until, after reinforcing him for behaviour that comes nearer and nearer to what we actually want, when we say, 'Hold the spoon', he puts his hand on the spoon with his fingers curling round it. Then we would go on to teach him to pick it up.

Shaping is one way of teaching a child to do new things, and it can be very useful, but it does have some drawbacks. First, it is very slow, though it can be usefully combined with other teaching methods. Second, although we choose to reinforce the child for something she does pretty often, we are at first dependent on her doing it of her own accord. It would be possible, for example, for Kevin never actually to pick up the spoon at all. This is in fact what happened when some nurses, using shaping, tried to teach a child to use a spoon: they got as far as I have described, with the child's hand resting on the spoon, but could get no further. So they went on to use prompting, which is what we are going to look at now.

Prompting

Prompting means helping the child to do the action – guiding her through it, then reinforcing her so that she will be more willing to try to do the action herself. This perhaps highlights the difference between reinforcement and reward. A reward is usually given for a virtuous action whereas reinforcement is given for an action that we want to encourage. If we help a child to do something, we may feel she hardly deserves a reward since she was hardly responsible for the action; but reinforcement is given so that she will be more likely to try to do it another time.

There are three kinds of prompts: the first, and most important, is *physical* prompting, the second prompting by *gesture*, the third *verbal* prompting. Very important too are the concrete, or structural, prompts that we can provide to help things along.

1. *Physical prompts*

In physical prompting we guide the child, using our hands to move her limbs, to do the action we want her to learn. In this way she herself will begin to feel, through the movements of her own body, how she should do the action; and because she is reinforced for the completed action she is the more eager to do it the next time.

Prompting is a good method to use for teaching a child to feed herself. Christine enjoys her food and can feed herself with her fingers, but she cannot manage a spoon and up till now has had to be fed all her meals. Christine is seated at the table, wearing an enveloping bib, with her plate in front of her, a suitable-sized spoon on the right-hand side (she is right-handed). Some food that she loves is put on her plate and a spoonful of it is ready in the spoon. We put her hand round the handle of the spoon and, holding our hand round hers, guide the spoon to her mouth, into it, tip the food off the spoon into her mouth and guide the spoon out of her mouth and back on to the plate. Since the food is something she likes the food itself is the reinforcer. When she has finished that mouthful we try again with another spoonful.

To take another example, we could use prompting to teach a child to sit down on request. So if this is what we want to teach Alec, we make sure we have a good supply of whatever is reinforcing for him — say, pieces of apple and cornflakes. We break the apple up into small bits (each quarter would be cut into about six pieces) and we take them and Alec to a chair that he can sit down on easily. We stand him with his back to the chair, say, 'Sit down Alec', gently push him down to sit on the chair, and immediately, as soon as his bottom touches the chair seat, praise him — 'Clever boy, Alec! That *is* good!' and at the same time pop a piece of apple or a cornflake into his mouth. In a few moments, when he has finished chewing and swallowing, we might stand him up and do the same thing two or three times more. Gradually we should find him becoming more ready to sit down of his own accord when we ask him to.

Teaching an action to a child in this way is not at all the same as just 'doing it for her'. Although at this point we are making the action happen, the child is also going through it, and is feeling the pattern of the movement in her own body, which leads on to her doing it eventually without help.

Physical prompting may be used on any part of the child's body — head, arms, legs, shoulders — or to move the whole child from one place to another, for example in teaching her to respond to the words 'Come here'. Prompting can also be used on smaller parts such as fingers, though this is more awkward and fiddly.

2. *Prompting by gesture*

Gestures can help children to understand what we want them to do, especially children who are attentive to other people. We often use gestures along with words, to make our meaning clear. For instance, we would point to the chair, or pat the seat, at the same time telling Alec to 'Sit down'. Later on we may have to be careful not to use too many gestures, if we want to be sure that the child really understands what we say: quite often children who have been thought to understand everything said to them are found to be responding more to the gestures that have always accompanied the words than to the words themselves.

Most gestures are made with the hand and arm, like pointing, but effective gestures can also be made with a jerk of the head or with 'eye-pointing' – glancing at or looking towards an object. These, especially, are the kind of gestures we may make without realizing it.

3. *Verbal prompts*

Verbal prompts tell the child in words what to do. Obviously they can only be useful with children who understand the message the words convey. Verbal prompts may be very general – 'Get dressed'; or, if this does not result in the action we hoped for it may be helpful to break down the sequence implied in that single instruction into a series of prompts: 'Open the cupboard; now get out your vest; put on your vest; now get out your pants', and so on.

These last two prompts, gestural and verbal, are often referred to as *cues*, because their function is more to indicate or hint to the child as to what she should do, rather than to produce it willy-nilly from her, as is the case with physical prompts. However, they all three perform a similar task in helping the child to do the action we want her to learn.

Setting the scene – using structural prompts

Up till now we have been discussing ways in which we can, by our own actions, help the child to do something new. Another way to help is by reorganizing or rearranging the surroundings.

For example, if Christine found it very difficult, as many children do, to scoop the food onto her spoon we could give her a bowl instead of a plate, or a special guard to fix onto the outside of her plate to make the scooping easier for her. Jack, who was learning to dress himself, was very much distracted by the sight of people walking up and down the corridor on the other side of his glass bedroom door: when a screen was put across he learned more quickly. Another boy, Timmy, who refused to drink out of a cup and always drank in small sips out of a spoon, gradually came round to drinking from a cup by being given, over a period of months, a series of spoons which gradually became deeper and the handle more curved until it was a cup. In these cases the children were helped to learn by changes in the objects around them, and this method can be used alongside any of the other prompts or other methods that you decide to use. These structural prompts are very important in that they are often quite simple to set up, and they can make it easier and quicker for the child to learn.

Here again we see the need for very small steps (each of Timmy's spoons was only fractionally different from the one before it) and, so that eventually Christine will be able to manage with an ordinary plate and Jack do without the screen, for fading (see below).

Fading the prompts

This is so important and so tricky it deserves a heading of its own.

As the child begins to learn what she has to do, through being prompted through the action, so she begins to take part in it, begins to put some effort into it and to take over the performance of some of the action. As she does so, her teacher *fades* out the prompt – the amount the teacher is contributing to the action – by just enough to allow the child to do as much as she can and will, but still ensuring that the action is successfully completed. This is amazingly difficult. It demands constant alertness and sensitivity on our part to the changing pattern of the child's response, so that we neither persist with iron grip in pushing her through movements which she could to some extent do on her own; nor make the opposite mistake of relaxing and releasing our prompts before the child has really taken over the action, so that the spoon (or whatever) clatters to the floor and the action grinds to a halt half-way through.

Fading physical prompts means that a prompt that was initially given firmly is given a little more lightly, then more lightly still, then more lightly again, and so on until we are not actually touching the child but still keep our hands over and very close to her; at the slightest sign of hesitation or difficulty we are there to help the action to completion. This method of keeping our hands very close to the child but not touching her is called *shadowing*.

Fading gestural and verbal prompts goes in much the same way. Gestures become less emphatic, and shorter; what was a rigidly pointing finger becomes a casual wave, and then less even than that. Verbal prompts, instructions or words, become shorter – 'Say "Good morning"' becomes 'Say "Good morn' ..."' then 'Say "Good mor' ..."' until it is only 'Say "G' ..."' – or it can become fainter, being said in a quieter and quieter voice until it is hardly a whisper.

The eventual aim of all prompting is that the child shall be able to do the action independently. This is achieved by very gradual fading of the prompts, and by never fading them so quickly that the child fails to complete the action. If in spite of all our efforts the child does falter this shows that we have been trying to fade the prompts too quickly, and that the child is not yet ready to take over so much of the action. We should at once go back, not necessarily to the beginning but to the level of prompt we were using just before the child faltered. And we should remember to fade the prompt more slowly this time.

Most problems seem to come from prompts being faded too

quickly. On the other hand we should always be on the alert to notice whether the child is able to do just a little more herself.

Breaking down an activity into small steps

When setting out to teach a child an activity she finds rather complicated it is usually best to break it down into a series of very small steps and teach one step at a time. If you think about Christine learning to spoon-feed herself, this involves picking up the spoon, pushing it into the food so that some food goes into it, raising it to her lips without turning it upside down, putting the bowl of the spoon into her mouth, tipping the food off the bowl of the spoon into her mouth, taking the spoon out of her mouth and returning it to her plate. Seven steps, and tipping up the plate to scrape the food together hasn't been included.

The important point is to make sure that the steps are really small enough. It is easy for us, because we are so used to doing these tasks, to underestimate how difficult they are for somebody who is learning them for the first time. I never realized what a complicated task it was to put on a cardigan until I saw my small daughter struggling with it. Tying a single knot seemed a simple process until I started teaching Philip (see page 87) to do it. So we break the task into as small steps as we possibly can. No harm is done if they are too small – the child just whizzes through a couple at a time – but if they are too large she may fail to learn and everyone gets discouraged. If your teaching stops working and the child fails to learn there are two questions you should first ask yourself: one, are the reinforcers really effective? two, are the steps in the task small enough?

When the task has been broken down the child can be taught first one step, then another, and then the two steps can be *chained* (or joined) together. *Forward chaining* involves teaching the child the first step first, and then chaining that to the second step, and so on.

Backward chaining

We often, however, prefer to use backward chaining which means teaching the *last* step *first*. This may sound odd, but the point is that the child becomes skilled first at the step that leads immediately to the completion of the task and so to reinforcement. When she has learnt this and does it easily, we then teach the preceding step that leads on to the last which she has already mastered, and then rapidly to reinforcement. In every case the likelihood of reinforcement is clearly before her, and this seems to help her to learn.

In the case of Christine learning to feed herself, if we taught her by forward chaining we would first teach her to pick up the spoon: there would then be quite a long gap before she received the reinforcement of eating the food. If we used backward chaining we would prompt her, without making any demands on her, right through the task until she got to the point where the food should be tipped into her mouth: we would relax the prompt at that point first, expecting that as she would be eager to get the food she would now be most willing to put in some effort of her own. When she was able to do this part of the task we would next relax the prompt just as the spoon reached her lips, so that now Christine would have to do some of the new step of putting the spoon into her mouth, following this with the familiar and well-learnt step of tipping the food into her mouth and enjoying the reinforcement – the food.

You may already have noted that on page 66 I spoke of returning the spoon to the plate, not tipping the food into Christine's mouth, as the last step. But as the food is the reinforcer, tipping it into the mouth is the step preceding reinforcement and it is the one we have to teach first. In fact it is often quite difficult to teach a child, who learns pretty well to take the spoon to her mouth, to return the spoon to the plate, presumably because the reinforcement – the next mouthful – is at that time so far away. She will often simply drop the spoon unless we are there to control it. It may be that taking the spoon to the mouth and returning it to the plate should be regarded as two separate tasks, and separate reinforcements could be earned for each. (Feeding is discussed in greater detail in chapter 11.)

The main points

1. We set out to teach the child something only just beyond what she is doing now.

2. Shaping involves reinforcing the child for doing something that gradually gets closer and closer to what we want her to learn.

3. Prompting means helping the child to perform the action and then reinforcing her for her part in the completed action.

4. There are three kinds of prompts: physical prompts, gestures and words (the last two are also often referred to as *cues*).

5. Setting the scene – structural prompts – can make the learning easier and quicker for the child.

6. Prompts should be minimal – only as much as is needed to ensure that the child performs the action.

7. Prompts should be very gradually faded as the child learns the task and takes it over.

8. A complicated task is easier to learn if it is broken down into very small steps, which are taught separately and then chained together.

9. Backward chaining – teaching the last step first and moving backwards in the chain – is often a good way of teaching.

Some practice problems

1. Try prompting another member of the family to do something – wash their hands, peel a potato, slice bread, kick a football, knit, anything.

2. Pretend that you are unable to do something, and get somebody else to prompt you to do it. (Don't forget the reinforcers!)

In each case try gradually fading the prompts.

3. Take some small, everyday task and break it down into small steps. Would it be best taught by forward or backward chaining?

*4. What structural prompts could you imagine using to teach a child to:
   (a) hang her coat on its own hook amongst other family hooks;
   (b) do up buttons;
   (c) recognize the tea-bag canister among a row of identical but named canisters (Tea, Sugar, Rice, etc.);
   (d) butter a slice of bread.

6. Imitation: Learning by Copying

Young children learn a good deal by imitating what they see other people do, and it is a particularly useful way of learning complicated skills. However, the ability to imitate is one that many children with learning disabilities lack. So we teach it to them.

To teach imitation we use methods discussed in the previous chapters, plus the new one of *modelling*. We ourselves do – model – the action to be imitated, *prompt* the child to do it, and *reinforce* her for her prompted response. Gradually, as she begins to be more ready to reproduce the modelled action, we *fade* the prompts until eventually she will imitate the model without any prompting.

After taking a baseline, and finding that she imitates very little or not at all, we start by teaching the child to imitate large, simple movements such as putting a brick in a cup, or raising arms out sideways: the reason for choosing these actions is chiefly that they are easy ones to prompt. If there is another person available it is very helpful to have him or her stand behind the child and act as prompter. The teacher stands (or sits) directly in front of the child, says, 'Do this', and models the action – for example, arms out sideways; the prompter then lifts the child's arms out to the side and the teacher instantly reinforces her. Then they try again, and after a few attempts the teacher waits for the child to hold the position herself for a moment before giving the reinforcement; later the prompter uses gradually less and less energy, as he feels the child doing more herself, until a light touch is all that is needed. Finally, when the teacher models the movement and says, 'Do this', the child produces a fair copy of the movement.

When the teacher is satisfied that the child can imitate one movement she moves on to another. This is an important step, because until now we cannot be sure that the child understands that the words 'Do this' mean 'Do whatever I do'; she may at this stage understand it to mean 'Do this particular action' (in this example, 'Raise your arms sideways'). Not until the child will attend to the modelled action, whatever it is, and then reproduce it, is it clear that she understands that she should imitate, not just that she should perform a particular action. This is rather different from responding to particular words, as discussed in the previous chapter, when the words 'Sit down' always meant, 'Carry out the particular action of sitting'. Now what is meant is, 'Be ready to do whatever you see done in front of you'. Again, because we are teaching the child to imitate, if she spontaneously, without being told 'Do this', raises her arms sideways, we do not reinforce her. We are not trying to teach her to raise her arms sideways: we are trying to teach her to do, when told, whatever she sees done. For the same reason it does not matter that the actions we ask her to do are ones which are not very useful like raising her arms out sideways; at the moment we are not trying to teach her a useful action, we are trying to teach her to imitate.

Having taught the child to imitate one movement, we teach her another: preferably a quite different one, like stepping on a box. Then we ask her to imitate the two movements whenever we make them, in a mixed-up order. Then we may teach another movement, and include it in with the others, and so on. When she has learned to imitate several large movements we go on to more complex ones (pick up a waste-paper basket and carry it across the room), or smaller movements, say, of the hands. As the child learns to imitate several movements we usually find that she needs less and less teaching on each one, until eventually she imitates without prompting the first time we do a new movement. When this happens the child has developed a *set* to imitate.

The development of an *imitative set* is of immense value for teaching a child actions that are difficult to prompt and many things are learned more easily through imitation: washing and drying dishes, how to behave in public, mouth-washing and gargling, road safety, table-top games, and so on. For children who may be helped by learning one of the sign systems (this applies to those children who may develop speech as well as those who, because of some special disability such as deafness, may not) the ability to imitate is extremely important; we can prompt hands and fingers into the shape needed for making signs but teaching this is very much easier if the child herself can try to imitate the shape she sees.

Who to imitate

It has been found that people are more ready to imitate someone whom they admire and find sympathetic – a warm, loving friend whose actions bring her success rather than a cold unsympathetic teacher who apparently gets little fun out of anything. Parents, of course, have many of the qualifications of a good model. However, it may be a good idea to try using as the model someone more like the child we are teaching – another child, a favourite brother or sister perhaps. Because the model is nearer her own age, and a child like herself, the child may be more inclined to imitate what she sees this model do. We may then have a few trial runs in which the child-model is asked to imitate something, and is reinforced for what he or she does. This will help the child-pupil to realize that imitating other people's actions brings reinforcement, and may sharpen up her interest and willingness to take part. In fact children often enjoy this imitation-learning which can be made into a game for them (it is after all closely related to the game of 'Simon says').

Imitating the wrong things

I said at the beginning of this chapter that, although for most children imitation comes naturally, many children with learning disabilities do not readily learn to imitate. It is all the more puzzling and frustrating then that they may be found to imitate in very specific ways: they can pick up the undesirable behaviours of others, especially of other children – head-banging, self-slapping, swearing, and so on. Why this happens, when they seem to have so much difficulty in imitating the things we would like them to, is not clear but they may see this behaviour as having the kind of spin-off that they would like: the head-banger is quickly attended to, the swearer elicits a shock-horror reaction from bystanders, the child showing these behaviours is the focus of all eyes. In other cases the imitation may result from curiosity – the child watches the self-slapper and tries slapping herself to see what it feels like.

Seeing a child pick up behaviours which she has not shown before can be very dismaying. Ideally we might prefer that she did not encounter children with these behaviours, but it may not always be possible for her to avoid them. In some cases, especially where it seems that the child was experimenting with the behaviour, it may simply die out; in others, particularly if the child finds that she gets something out of it (it is reinforcing to her), we may have to try to tackle the problem. You can find some ideas on how to deal with problem behaviours, in particular swearing and to a lesser extent self-injury, in chapter 7.

Imitation is then a way in which the child can learn new skills. She may then need to learn one of two things connected with her new skill: either *generalization* or *discrimination*. I will discuss each of these in turn.

Generalization

The child may need to learn that a piece of behaviour learnt in one place, in the company of one person, working with one object, may apply equally well in another place, with another person, and another object; or in a number of places, with many people, and with a wide variety of objects. In this way she learns to *generalize* the action.

Suppose David's mother teaches him to drink from a cup. She always uses a particular yellow plastic cup that is David's own, and because at the beginning he was likely to make rather a mess she has always carried out her teaching in the kitchen with its lino floor. When David has learnt the task, his mother may find to her dismay that he will only drink in the kitchen, from the yellow cup, when she is there. He won't drink in his bedroom, or from a blue china mug, or when his uncle offers him a drink. This is a somewhat extreme example: it is unusual for a child to be quite so specific as to how she will drink. Nevertheless, there are plenty of examples in which a piece of behaviour which has been quite well learnt is so limited in its application as to be positively embarrassing. Simon, for example, learnt to use the toilet in his home, but that was the only one he would use; so his mother could never take him out for a day, or even for part of a day, because he adamantly refused to use any toilet but the one at home.

So the child may need to be taught to generalize what she learns. What we have to teach her, in fact, is that a piece of behaviour that is reinforced in one situation is likely to be reinforced in another. David needs to learn that if he enjoys a pleasant drink and a caress from his mother when he is in the kitchen he is equally likely to get both enjoyments if he drinks in the bedroom or dining-room; if he gets them from drinking from a yellow plastic cup he will also get them from drinking from a pink plastic cup or a yellow china cup. He may, of course, learn this or some of this of his own accord – many children do. But it is a good principle, when teaching children with learning disabilities, not to bank on their doing so. To be on the safe side, we should build generalization into our teaching programme.

For a start, it is always a good idea to teach the child in the place where, and with the people with whom, she is most likely to be. This is why it is no longer thought best for children to be taught, as a rule, by specially trained psychologists or teachers, in special laboratories, the things that they will mostly need to use at home (although there may be cases where this is necessary). They usually make better progress if they are taught at home. Even this, however, may not be enough, as we saw in the case of Simon and the toilet. We may need to ensure that the skill can be generalized to occur in different parts of the home or outside the home, in the presence of people other than the original teacher, and with a variety of suitable objects.

There are two ways we can make sure that this generalization takes place. We may teach the child in the normal way, expecting that she will have little difficulty in generalizing what she has learnt; then, if she does show some difficulty in other situations, we can be ready to help her relearn it. Many children will have relatively little difficulty in relearning, or learning to generalize, a skill. If, however, we realize that the child is likely to have difficulty in generalizing we should deliberately include it as part of her training. This happened with Simon. The difficulty Simon had had in generalizing from one toilet to another was taken into account when he was taught a new skill – buttoning; his teacher took care to vary the teaching situation from the start. She taught him buttoning in his bedroom, another child's bedroom, the bathroom or the passage; she, his mother and his father all took part in the teaching; he buttoned his pyjama jacket, an anorak, a coat belonging to another child, and his own shirt. In this way Simon learnt to do up buttons in many different circumstances; once he had learnt it he was able to do it whenever he needed to and not just in one particular set of conditions.

Discrimination

This is the other side of the coin. If a child must learn that some kinds of behaviour which are reinforced in one situation are also reinforced in others, she must also learn that there are some other kinds of behaviour which are reinforced only in certain specific situations; and she must learn to *discriminate* between these situations.

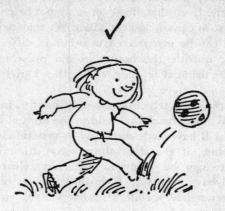

For instance, she must learn that it is all right to throw a ball but not all right to throw a pot plant or occasional table; it is all right to undress when she is going to bed, or to have a bath or a swim but not in the supermarket; it is all right to hug and kiss a member of her family when they meet, but not the policeman; she should clean her teeth with her toothbrush but not with anyone else's.

To teach discrimination we use the same methods discussed before: prompting if necessary, reinforcing the right responses and not reinforcing the wrong ones. In addition, we try to help the child to pick out and attend to the signals, the *cues*, that tell her whether or not reinforcement is likely. These cues, telling the child what sort of behaviour is expected of her (and therefore likely to be reinforced), may consist of a variety of things – a place, a person, something happening, a word or a sentence may all act as cues for a piece of behaviour. A red traffic light is a cue to stop, a green light one to go ahead. A strict teacher may be a cue to a child to behave sedately, an indulgent grandmother a cue to kick over the traces. A nearby chair plus a few friendly words from an adult may be a cue to a child to sit down (which is why we should be cautious about believing that she knows the meaning of the words 'Sit down';

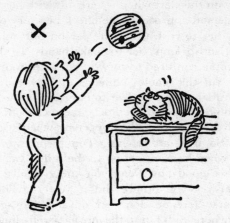

if a chair were in the vicinity she might, if we said, 'Go to bed', sit down just the same – the chair itself may be an important cue). The banging of a gong may be a cue to go to the dining-room, and the words 'Dinner is ready' may serve the same purpose.

Many of the cues to which we respond are complex and subtle: a slight chilliness in someone's manner can deter you from speaking to them, a person in a blue uniform with a yellow band round her hat walking along a pavement may cause you to park the car elsewhere. These sorts of cues are often difficult for the child with learning disabilities to pick up. She may at times fail to make the right response, not because she does not know how to do it, but because she didn't understand what was expected of her. We can help her to produce the kind of behaviour we want by making the cues very clear.

So if we want to teach her to play with balls outside, in the garden, the park or the beach but not inside the house, we keep *all* the balls, footballs, tennis balls, beach balls, outside in the garden shed or in a box outside the front door, and do not have any balls, not even fluffy ones or marbles, in the house. If she tends to greet all and sundry by flinging her arms round them we stay on the alert when we are out with her and when a non-family person approaches we check her very early on: we do not allow her to rush up to the person but hold her back, and then tell and prompt her to shake hands. In this way she does not become confused as to where the appropriate behaviour begins, but the whole sequence of how she should approach unfamiliar people is clear to her. Again, the cues which the child should attend to should be distinct from their background, and this is especially important when we are giving instructions. So, if we are teaching Tony, who cannot speak, to make a sign when he wants to go to the toilet, we don't say to him: 'That's-a-good-boy-Tony-you-know-what-you-have-to-do-don't-you-yes-you-do-we-did-it-yesterday-no-don't-do that-now-come-here-no-don't-sit-on-the-floor-get-up-yes-that's-good-where-did-I-put-the-oh-yes-well-done-give-me-your-hand-give-it-to-me-now . . .' Instead we get down to Tony's level, we make sure he is facing us, and then we say, 'Tony, do "toilet".' Just that.

Another important area in which we should make the cues very clear is that of the approval and disapproval that we show the child. Most children can get the message from a barely perceptible shake of the head or a murmured 'Good'; for the disabled child the message needs to be made more distinct.

Again (and providing we know the child is not one who reacts badly to warm enthusiasm, see page 37) we use as many different ways as we can think of to get the message across – words, voice, facial expression, the way we use our hands. A thumbs-up sign, plus a delighted voice saying, 'Tony, that's *terrific*', plus a wide smile and a pat on the back all emphasize that we are pleased. Tony is left in no doubt that he has done the right thing. Here, too, it is important for the approval-cue, and in its turn the disapproval cue, to be quite distinct from their background. If you look back at the 'verbal garbage' above you will see that there are in it three approval-cues and two disapproval-cues: but I doubt you noticed them.

Nor would Tony.

The main points

1. When we teach a child to imitate, we:
   say, 'Do this';
   model the action;
   prompt the child;
   reinforce her for the prompted response.

2. As the child begins to do some of the action, we gradually *fade* our prompt.

3. We start by teaching large simple movements.

4. It may help to have one person as model and reinforcer, a second person as prompter.

5. When one action has been learned we teach another: then give them in a mixed-up order.

6. From large simple movements we go on to more complex, or to finer movements (hands and fingers).

7. Imitation is useful for children learning language, either speech or a sign system.

8. Generalization means that a child who has learnt to do something in one situation can apply it in other situations.

9. Generalization may need to be taught by reinforcing what the child learns in many different situations.

10. Discrimination means that a child learns that she should do something in certain situations, not in others.

11. We teach discrimination by reinforcing these things in the appropriate situations and not reinforcing them in others.

12. The cues that tell a child that her actions are likely to be reinforced should be very clear.

Some practice problems

*1. Can you think of two or three things that you or any member of your family have learned by imitation?

*2. Is there any other way you might have been taught these things?

*3. Can you think of any behaviour of a non-disabled child (of your own or someone else's) which was learnt in a very specific situation and did not easily generalize?

 4. How was this difficulty got over?

*5. What are the cues that tell us to:
   (*a*) Put on a mackintosh;
   (*b*) Drive on a certain side of a road;
   (*c*) Raise our voice;
   (*d*) Give over money;
   (*e*) Get out of bed?
   (There may be more than one possible cue to each action.)

7. Learning Not To

This book is mainly concerned with ways of teaching children new skills. Children with learning disabilities need to learn all sorts of useful and interesting things and the main focus of our efforts is to help them to do so. Like other children, however, they may sometimes exhibit behaviours that we would rather they didn't – bad behaviours – and that we want to help them to get rid of.

Getting rid of bad behaviours may be important for several reasons. First, the behaviours may hinder the child herself in learning new skills that would be useful to her – for instance, if she spends much of her time rocking it may be difficult, until she stops rocking enough to be able to pay attention, to teach her more useful things such as putting on her socks or playing with a toy. Second, the behaviours may upset other people – interfering with their belongings, disturbing the peace, making it difficult for them to get on with everyday life, messing up their surroundings, making a lot of extra work for them, and so on. The disadvantage to the child herself and the disturbance to other people can also interact; sometimes the child, through her bad behaviour, puts people off her so that they are unwilling to spend time with her and teach her. For all these reasons she may need to be taught that there are some things that she should not do. This chapter is about ways of teaching this.

In the ordinary way, when children do something wrong they may be punished, and the punishment will usually consist of something seen as unpleasant – a scolding, docking of pocket-money, not being allowed out to play, or whatever. For many people 'punishment' automatically includes, amongst other things, retribution: the child herself should suffer to some extent for the wrong she has done. Where children with learning disabilities are concerned, retribution does *not* come into it. We are not out to make them suffer; we want to help them to live more enjoyable lives. Since this may involve teaching them to unlearn or give up some behaviours, what we do is look for and use methods which, *when they follow a behaviour, make it less likely that that behaviour will occur in the future*.

You can see that this definition is the exact opposite of the definition of reinforcement on page 28. You can see too that it says nothing about what might be used to bring about the lessening of the behaviour. No assumptions are made about that. Indeed, some things that we might think of as unpleasant, such as a scolding, may not reduce a behaviour at all, while some other action that seems very mild, like looking away from the child for a few seconds, or putting her in her toy-strewn bedroom for a few minutes (see the example of Tim on page 95) may succeed in doing so. As with reinforcement, the crucial question for those using behavioural methods is: what effect does our method have on the behaviour? We are not interested in making the child suffer for her misdeeds; our concern is to see her bad behaviour lessen.

There are two or three things we can do as a start.

Trying to understand the behaviour

Just as with other kinds of behaviour, the first thing we should do is to make some observations, looking carefully at exactly what the problem behaviour is, when it happens, who else is likely to be involved in it, and so on. Once we have done that it may be useful to pause for a moment and ask ourselves some questions. What is the point of this behaviour? Can we see why the child is doing it? What does she get out of it? What does it do for her? We may then be able to see a way of helping her to get whatever it is that she seems to want in a better way.

'What are you trying to tell us?'

Trying to understand the behaviour is particularly important for children who cannot talk, or perhaps have great difficulty in communicating at all. We may find that the behaviour is the only way the child has to let us know what she feels about some things. For example, Colin would bite his hand, sometimes breaking the skin. Observation showed that he was most likely to do this when he was asked to do a new task, especially one that was more difficult than the tasks he had been doing before. He could not speak, and the biting seemed to be his way of trying to convey the message, 'I can't cope with this'. So he was given a small card with a big cross on it, and taught that when he showed this to the person working with him the task he was working on would be removed and he would be offered something less taxing to do. At the same time the tasks he was given were reconsidered, and the jump in the level of difficulty in any new task for him was made smaller, so that he was not so distressed by it. After some time Colin learned to use the card when he needed to, and did not bite his hand so often.

Similarly, children who cannot talk sometimes have tantrums apparently when they cannot get something they want or, alternatively, when they are prevented from doing something they want to do. In both cases, as with Colin, we need to teach the child a way of communicating her wishes other than by throwing a tantrum. There are a number of ways in which we can approach this. Probably most people would think first of teaching the child to make a sign; although we could make use of any gesture or sign the child makes it may be better, in order that she will be understood by people other than those in her immediate surroundings, to teach her a sign from one of the accepted sign systems. The one most widely used in this country for children with learning disabilities is the Makaton Vocabulary, a language programme which provides a small basic signed vocabulary specifically chosen to enable basic communication (see Appendix 2). So if we think that the most usual reason that Sonia throws a tantrum is that she wants a drink, we would teach her the sign for 'drink', using modelling (see page 70), prompting and fading the prompts (see pages 61–6).When she made the sign (even if at first with help from us) we would give her a drink (this is the reinforcer). If it was not possible to teach her to sign we could give her pictures, or photos, of the things she most often wanted, which she would be taught to show, or point to, when she wanted one of these things. Derek, who learned how to use pictures of several things – a drink, toilet, biscuit, bed – used to carry the pictures on a chain round his neck, and would pick out and point to whichever one he wanted at that moment. Some children, although unable to speak, have been able to learn to use written words to indicate their needs; although this is unusual, if it can be done it offers a flexible communication system for the child.

What we are trying to do here is to give the child a better way of expressing her needs than by throwing a tantrum (or in Colin's case, by biting his hand). Whenever we can we respond by giving whatever has been signed for. Inevitably, though, the time comes, as it may with any other form of request, when the child cannot have the thing she has asked for, and the request has to be refused. Nevertheless, the fact that we have understood the request means that we can acknowledge the child's need, we can show her that we know what she is asking for and that we are sorry that on this occasion she cannot be given it; her request is treated with respect. David, who loved going for walks and used to hit people when he wanted to go out, was taught to use the sign 'Out', and at first when he did so he was always taken out. Later he had to learn that this was not always possible; his teacher told him that she realized that he wanted to go out, that she was sorry that there was no one to go out with him at the moment but that he would go out as soon as this could be managed. David was not very pleased at this but he did not go back to hitting people, and he *was* taken out as soon as this was possible.

Cheering things up

Sometimes our observations may suggest that the child has a rather dreary lifestyle, with little of interest going on in it, or with little reinforcement coming her way. In this case it may be that her bad behaviours are a way of protesting, or they may simply be a way of occupying herself. So one of the first things we might do would be to make a real effort to improve her quality of life. In an American hospital ward for teenage girls the amount of aggression they vented on each other dropped dramatically when all the girls were routinely, once an hour, given some small titbit to eat. I am not suggesting that we should necessarily dish out food, but it might be that more cuddles, attention paid when it is not demanded, little treats or outings introduced into the daily routine, would in themselves have a good effect on the behaviour. Similarly, extra activities, whether they are teaching sessions or just recreational, may help – there is no doubt that children with learning disabilities can become bored. When they have more to do some of the bad behaviours may become less apparent.

Going about it

Changing the surroundings

One of the most straightforward things we can do is to help to avoid, or prevent, bad behaviours by altering the child's surroundings. Many parents of young children do this as a matter of course: for example, dealing with the children's tendency to break small objects and ornaments by clearing them away into the attic until the children are older. In the same way Paul, who would pull the hair of any child he sat next to, was seated well away from other children in the classroom, while, as an extra precaution, the other children's hair was tied up. Of course, this didn't teach Paul not to pull other children's hair; but it did allow him to learn other things and to be reinforced for what he did, whereas previously so much of his time had been taken up with hair-pulling. As Paul began to enjoy what he was learning and the reinforcement he was getting for it, it was possible to move him gradually nearer to the other children without his constantly pulling their hair.

Avoiding the behaviour in this way makes things easier for

everyone else involved, and can allow other kinds of behaviour to emerge, but it does not actually teach them to the child; so it is often combined with other methods such as prompting or shaping, or, in Paul's case, DRO, which we mentioned earlier (see page 44).

Differential Reinforcement of Other kinds of behaviour – DRO

This is one of the most positive ways of tackling bad behaviours. We do it, not by attacking the bad behaviour itself, but by building up other, good, behaviours to take its place. If possible we go for other behaviours which, while the child is engaged in them, make it impossible for her to do the bad behaviour at the same time – the two are incompatible. In some cases it has taken time and ingenuity to get this right. Carol, a nearly blind girl with very severe learning disabilities, was further damaging her sight by constantly poking her fingers in her eyes. As she was very fond of loud squeaky sounds she was given a switch to press which, so long as she kept her hand on it, played a tape of these sounds. Carol loved this, but then found that she could press the switch with one hand and still poke her eyes with the other. So the machinery was altered so that she now had two switches which had to be pressed at the same time to make the tape play. Surely now the eye-poking and sound-playing were incompatible – she could not have them both at the same time? We had underestimated Carol. She learnt to operate one of the switches with her elbow, which meant that again she could have the tape playing and still have a hand available to poke her fingers in her eye. Finally, with all the technical wizardry at our command, the switches were designed so that they would only work if Carol pressed them with the fingertips of both hands; at last this did make it impossible for her to poke her eyes while playing the tape. After this, although she did not alto- gether stop eye-poking, at least there were many times when she was pressing the switches and listening to the sounds she enjoyed and could not at the same time poke her fingers in her eyes.

In many cases DRO is a much simpler affair. If a child has a particular bad behaviour that we want to help her get over, we may tackle this by reinforcing her for just not doing it – reinforcing her when she is doing anything else *but* the behaviour. Chrissie's parents gave her lots of reinforcement whenever she was *not* crying (see page 89) and Trevor was reinforced when he ate without gobbling or using his fingers (see page 161). In another case Philip's parents asked for help with his habit of coming into their bed every night: it was suggested that, besides taking him back to his own bed whenever he came to the parents' room, for every night that he did not come to their room he should be given a star to be put on a chart, and when he had (the parents decided) four stars he would be taken to the toy shop to buy a new toy. So Philip's not-coming-in was reinforced, and this resulted in an immediate and dramatic cessation of interrupted nights for his parents.

As we said earlier, one of the main aims of a DRO programme is to build up a positive behaviour to take the place of the bad behaviour. Where this happens, the positive behaviour often becomes enjoyable to the child, either because the new skill learned is an enjoyable one or because other reinforcers, for example social reinforcers, take over. It can then be possible to fade out the reinforcers that were used to build up the behaviour. Ann (see page 45) got tokens, which she would later exchange for the CD she hankered for, for doing the things her mother asked her to do; previously she had usually refused to do what she was asked, so when she began carrying out these requests with alacrity her mother found this very pleasant, and quite naturally found herself responding more warmly to Ann. Ann in her turn liked this, and was the more ready to comply with her mother's friendly requests. As her mother said later on, 'We're such good friends now'.

DRO is a positive, gentle way of dealing with bad behaviours. Whatever method we use it is always worth trying to combine tackling the bad with building up a good behaviour alongside. This will help to ensure, first, that the child has a chance of getting the enjoyment (reinforcement) that she needs, and of which she may to some extent be deprived by our method of treating the bad behaviour; second, that she makes progress in positive things as well as learning not to do the bad things; and third, that concentration on what she should do as well as on what she should not will help to speed up the reduction in her present misbehaviour and, which is very important, make it less likely that new forms of it will appear in the future.

Extinction

In the last section we looked at ways in which we can use reinforcement to build up behaviours we want to counter those we do not. Sometimes, however, we can find that reinforcement has regularly (or irregularly) followed behaviours that we do not want at all. Nobody does this deliberately; nevertheless it can happen. When we realize what is happening, we may decide to change tack, and that in future we will not reinforce the behaviour; if we stick to this, the behaviour should in time disappear. This approach is called *extinction*: the reinforcer which has customarily followed the behaviour no longer does so; without the reinforcer to keep it going, the behaviour should die out (extinguish).

Chrissie was a bright little 6-year-old who tyrannized her entire family by crying. She cried a great deal of every day, especially when she had to go to school (although she enjoyed school), at any time when her mother had to leave her, when her father returned from work, when visitors came, when she went to a party, if she didn't go to a party. Her parents had consulted numerous doctors and psychiatrists, who had said Chrissie was 'deeply disturbed'. Chrissie continued to cry and her parents were at their wits' end. Careful observation showed that when Chrissie cried her concerned and loving parents showered her with attention, asked her what was the matter, begged her to tell them if anything unpleasant had happened, and so on and so on. The psychologist discussed with them the fact that Chrissie seemed to be getting reinforcement (attention) when she cried. They agreed that in future they would take no notice of her when she cried. We should not underestimate the difficulty for the parents in carrying out this programme: you can perhaps imagine for yourself how hard it would be to turn your back on your pathetically sobbing little 6-year-old when every fibre of your being is crying out to scoop her up and comfort her. However, perhaps because Chrissie's crying was wrecking family life and they were desperate, Chrissie's parents faithfully carried out the programme and ignored her crying. At the same time they strongly reinforced Chrissie – gave her a great deal of warm, loving attention – whenever she was *not* crying (this being an example of DRO, which we've just discussed).

What followed was fairly typical of what happens when extinction is used. To begin with, Chrissie's crying got worse. Finding that she could no longer get her mother's attention by just crying Chrissie first cried harder, then screamed distressingly; when her mother still did not turn round to her Chrissie beat her mother on the bottom with her fists; finally, as the time for school approached, Chrissie rushed up into the bathroom and made herself sick. At this point Chrissie's mother rang up the psychologist, and it was decided that, as Chrissie did not seem to be ill, she was to be taken calmly to school. Chrissie found that in spite of her intensified efforts she did not manage to get the reinforcement she had previously been accustomed to get for her crying, but that she did get it for other things – chatting with her family, drawing pictures, talking about her pet rabbit, helping to lay the table, going out for walks. So she still got attention, but not now for crying. This was quite a change. It may be that previously she did not get so much attention for the other things, that in the times when she was not crying the family thankfully got on with their own lives and tended to leave her alone. Now, though, she found that if crying did not bring her attention, other more ordinary activities did, and she began to cry less and less until, about three months later, she was a very different, cheerful, self-reliant, little girl who went happily off to school in the morning.

That her mother did not give in when Chrissie intensified her crying, and never attended to her crying once the programme was under way, was of enormous importance for the success of the project. If her mother had given in Chrissie would have learnt that, even if 'normal' crying no longer brought her reinforcement, she could still get the attention she craved by crying longer or harder. Once she had learnt this it would have been very much more difficult to treat the crying by extinction as Chrissie would have got the idea that, even if the present level of her crying did not bring the reinforcement, she only had to do it a little bit more – and a little bit more – and a little bit more – and sooner or later the adults would crack and reinforcement would be hers. If Chrissie successfully learnt this lesson she might learn to persist with, or to intensify, her crying to the point where it became impossible for her parents to hold out any longer.

So it is an important rule that, where a bad behaviour is being treated by extinction, it must *never* be reinforced.

As we have seen, when Chrissie's mother first embarked on her extinction programme, and withdrew the reinforcement – attention – that Chrissie had been used to getting for her crying, Chrissie cried harder. It is quite usual for a child's behaviour to get worse before it gets better when it is treated by extinction. Obviously it is important for parents to know this, before they start on the programme. If her mother had not known beforehand that Chrissie would probably cry harder at first she would have been quite likely to drop the programme like a hot potato saying, 'I tried that and it made her worse.' As it was, she knew that this worsening of Chrissie's behaviour was to be expected, and she was prepared to persist.

In Chrissie's case, where the problem was crying, and in the case of many other undesirable but fairly harmless behaviours, extinction is a useful treatment method. In some cases, however, as when the bad behaviour consists of serious self-injury, or aggression to other children, extinction may not be a good method, simply because of the fact that the behaviour can be expected to get worse before it improves. We would not be justified in allowing a child to do serious damage either to herself or to other children, even if we felt confident that later the damaging behaviour would lessen. By that time irreparable harm might have been done. In these cases other kinds of treatment must be found.

Extinction can be used to treat problem behaviours by withholding almost any kind of reinforcement, except those the child makes within herself (see page 93). It is especially suitable for those children who enjoy provoking adults, and who seem to get reinforcement from the upset they cause, and from the distress, irritation or anger of the adults around them (see page 34).*

Once we realize that anger does not necessarily discourage the child's bad behaviour, but actually increases it, a programme can be worked out in which we will no longer react angrily, or will not, probably, react at all, to the child's bad behaviour. How easy it will be to carry out this programme is another matter: it is not always easy to remain unflinchingly calm while a child spits accurately in your eye or pushes over every item of furniture in the room. However, once again, if we decide to apply extinction it is most important that we should be consistent about it: if, goaded beyond endurance, we eventually give the child the attention she has been working for she will realize that persistence pays dividends and be encouraged to persist even more.

---

* That scolding may be a reinforcer and, if it is withheld, the unacceptable behaviour may die out (extinguish) is not an entirely new idea. Here, in a passage written in 1815, the couple, who have just got engaged to each other, are a man, and a girl half his age.

'Mr Knightley. You always called me Mr Knightley.'

'I remember once calling you "George", in one of my amiable fits, about ten years ago. I did it because I thought it would offend you; but as you made no objection, I never did it again.'

Jane Austen, *Emma*, chapter 17.

Extinction is a powerful method of getting rid of patterns of behaviour. It is important to realize that it can work on good as well as on bad behaviour. If we have been reinforcing a child for something we want her to do, and then stop reinforcing her for it, that piece of behaviour is likely to die out eventually. This is particularly likely to happen if we change suddenly from giving a lot of reinforcement to giving none at all. So in the case of good behaviour we need to guard against the possibility of extinction by going from a consistent to an every-now-and-again kind of reinforcement (see page 38). The reinforcement can become more and more infrequent but we should try to make sure that we continue to reinforce the good behaviour, at least occasionally. There is an exception to this – where what the child is learning is in itself reinforcing: for instance, if you teach a child to read, or to ride a bicycle, once she has learnt the activity thoroughly the Smarties and expressions of delight will not be needed; she enjoys reading and cycling for their own sakes. But with other activities that are not in themselves reinforcing we need to be careful not to allow them to be extinguished for want of occasional reinforcement.

Time-out from positive reinforcement

Like extinction, this is a method which relies on the management of reinforcement. When we use extinction, the reinforcement that has usually followed the behaviour no longer does so: when we use time-out, the reinforcement goes on all the time but is interrupted if the behaviour occurs. When this method is used the child is ordinarily in a very enjoyable situation, getting a lot of reinforcement, until she behaves badly; then the reinforcement suddenly disappears. After a short time the reinforcement becomes available to her again, and only disappears if she behaves badly again.

Let's take an example. Alice is a little girl with severe learning disabilities who had a habit of smearing her own saliva on her hands and rubbing it all over her face. This doesn't sound very bad but it made Alice smell unpleasant, so that people tended to avoid coming near her. Her teacher decided to try to stop her smearing her face. Alice loved being tickled, so tickling was used as the reinforcement. The teacher would play with and tickle Alice continuously: as soon as Alice smeared saliva over her face the teacher stopped the tickling and only began it again five seconds after Alice had stopped smearing. In time Alice smeared her face less, she smelled more pleasant, and people were more willing to do things with her.

Time-out can be used whenever the reinforcer is one we can control. Time-out cannot be used where the reinforcer is impossible for another person to control, such as the reinforcement gained from the feeling of tongue-rolling or lip-smacking; luckily this sort of reinforcer is pretty unusual. If a child is fond of one particular toy, time-out might mean removing the toy for a short time whenever she behaved badly. TV was used as a reinforcer with a little boy who sucked his fingers until they were raw, especially when he was watching TV: every time his fingers went to his mouth the TV set was switched off for ten seconds. Another boy, Don, who at 12 years old had severe learning and physical disabilities, was very fond of music and his mother used to switch on the radio when she went into his bedroom in the morning. She said that day after day he was very difficult to dress as he would become silly and giggly and deliberately stiffen his arms and legs as she was trying to get them through the sleeves and legs of his clothes. So it was decided that when he did this he would be timed-out from his reinforcement – the radio was switched off for fifteen seconds. So long as Don cooperated in the dressing process the music-reinforcer was always there; as soon as he became difficult he lost it. Don learnt that it was more fun for him – he was able to listen to the music he loved without interruption – if he cooperated, and his mother found him progressively easier to dress.

Misbehaviour at meal-times can be treated by time-out from the meal – if the child is very keen on her food; we would not get far if we timed her out from a meal she didn't want much anyway. Trevor was very, very fond of his food and would eat practically anything. So anxious was he to get his food that he would gulp it down, cramming one mouthful in on top of another and using his fingers to eat with instead of his knife and fork. So each of these things was treated by time-out from the meal – his plate was taken away for ten seconds each time one of them occurred. He quite quickly learnt to swallow one mouthful before putting in another and not to use his fingers.

The time-out is kept as short as possible, partly because we do not want to deprive the child of reinforcement for any longer than we have to, and partly because it has been found that long periods of time-out actually work less well. It seems that with long periods the child may forget what it was for, what the behaviour was that occasioned it; it is then less likely that she will try to avoid the behaviour that led to the time-out because she does not associate the two. So long periods of time-out may be less likely to lead to an improvement in the behaviour than shorter ones. As a rule of thumb, we can usually end the time-out and restore the reinforcement about 5–10 seconds after the behaviour, for which the time-out was imposed, stops. So the finger-sucker learned to take his fingers out of his mouth quite quickly when the TV was switched off, and Don soon learned to relax his arms and legs when the music disappeared. Trevor's food-snatching usually resulted in his getting a mouthful of food before his plate was removed, so it was necessary to wait for him to finish the mouthful, and then wait another ten seconds or so, before his plate was given back to him.

Time-out can be used with many kinds of reinforcers, and can be used effectively where the reinforcers are social ones – attention, praise, smiles, hugs and kisses, or the social situation of being with other people. So time-out may be given in different ways, depending on exactly what the social reinforcer is. If the child very much enjoys an adult's attention, time-out may consist of the adult moving away from the child, or turning his back on her, or even just turning away his head.

Then when the child's behaviour has stopped for a few seconds the adult turns back to her.

So far I have not talked about the kind of time-out from positive reinforcement that consists, when the bad behaviour occurs, of the child's being put in a room on her own. At one time this kind of time-out was quite widespread but its use has diminished, over the years, mainly because of worries about possible abuse of the method, and the possibility of it leading to cruelty. These are serious concerns, and it is very important that this kind of time-out should not be used carelessly. However, it may be a suitable method to use on occasion, especially when the child is very disruptive; apart from anything else, it can allow the situation to calm down. Tim, who had learning disabilities and autism, used to have tantrums in which he screamed and hit and kicked his mother. She decided that when he did this he would be put in his bedroom until he had calmed down and was quiet for thirty seconds. Tim's room was not at all unpleasant, it still had all his toys in it except his tape recorder which his mother removed when she left him in there. Over the weeks in which his mother put this programme into effect the number of tantrums Tim had went steadily down, he needed to go to his room less and less often, and he and his mother were able to have a happier relationship.

At this point perhaps a question which is often raised should be dealt with: if the child's bedroom is used as a time-out room will she come to hate it, and be afraid or unwilling to sleep in it? This seems to me an entirely reasonable worry; I can only say that neither I nor the other workers whom I have consulted have ever known this to happen. It may help to understand this if we realize that what we are doing is not punishing the child by putting her *in* a nasty place; instead, we are taking her *away* from a pleasurable situation. So going to her bedroom is not a matter of going to a horrid place, but of an interruption of whatever enjoyable things had been going on. So her bedroom is not frightening, and at bedtime is still, to her, her normal place for sleeping.

Using the child's bedroom as a place to cool off is quite common in many families with ordinary children ('You can come out when you can be friendly', my small grandson was told, and he did, about five minutes later), and it may also be helpful for some families with a learning-disabled child. Again, it is very important not to use long periods of time, such as half an hour or more. We need to remember that the method we are using is *time-out from positive reinforcement*, and if the time-out is quite short, the interruption of the reinforcement – the good time the child was having until the behaviour took place – seems more noticeable.

Time-out should never be used as an excuse for a bit of peace and quiet for us.

Brief restraint

The ways of dealing with bad behaviours that I have been discussing so far are the positive ones, changing the surroundings and managing reinforcement. These are the ones that I would always look to first, in that order. Sometimes, though, we may need to respond to and tackle the behaviour directly.

To many of us as children (myself among them) serious naughtiness was followed by a smack. Smacking has gone up and down in popularity over the years. The Victorians used the expression 'Spare the rod and spoil the child', but smacking has become much less acceptable – to some people now, entirely wrong. I suppose many parents, goaded by an infuriating child, will give vent to their feelings with a slap, and this may be the best we can say about it: smacking may be more a way of relieving the parents' feelings than of doing anything to improve the child's behaviour. There is not much evidence that smacking makes children good, and indeed there are some indications that a lot of smacking may make them worse.*

* J. & E. Newson, *The Extent of Physical Punishment in the UK*, APPROACH (Association for the Protection of All Children), London, 1989.

Some parents of children with learning disabilities have found this out for themselves.

'It stops her at the time but whether she really understands what it's for I don't know.'

'It works for the moment but it doesn't really alter his behaviour.'*

So smacking may be not only wrong in itself but also not a useful way to change behaviour, and I do not propose to discuss it further. There is, however, a way of responding to some behaviours that may be useful – brief restraint.

Sometimes a child's behaviour may be so frenetic that it is difficult to catch her attention sufficiently to use any of the other methods already discussed. Then we may hold her quite still for a few seconds, say, for a count of ten. After this we let go of her in order to get back to normal activities. The out-of-control behaviour is interrupted and the child has the chance to adopt another, quieter, behaviour. If, however, when we have released her, she misbehaves again, we hold her again in the same way, and we repeat this until when we release her she does not misbehave.

Andy's misbehaviour consisted of, amongst other things, kicking and hitting adults, and he would become quite over-wrought at these times. It was decided to try the use of restraint. The next time he hit someone his arms were calmly and firmly held. When he was released he hit out again and again he was held, and this sequence was carried out four times altogether before he behaved quietly when he was released. After two or three occasions like this Andy needed only one period of restraint following his misbehaviour – with that particular adult. Andy did not readily generalize his learning and had to learn afresh with several different people that whenever he hit or kicked, his arms would be held; he became calmer, and it was possible to go on to teach him some more interesting things.

* Janet Carr, *Young Children with Down's Syndrome* (see Appendix 3).

In using brief restraint we have to watch out for the possibility that it may be reinforcing; that, far from decreasing it may actually increase the behaviour. Just as expressions of anger may be reinforcing so, to a child who very much enjoys adult attention and closeness, restraint may be enjoyable. We try to guard against this by giving her little attention during the restraint, turning our heads away and not speaking to her (and, of course, looking for times when she is calm to give her plenty of attention and closeness). Here again our records are important. If they show the number of occurrences of the bad behaviour going up, then it is likely that, despite our efforts, the child is finding the restraint reinforcing. We had better look for something else.

Some special problems: swearing, masturbation and self-injury

Behavioural methods lay great stress on careful observation of each child, so that it is possible to judge what particular methods are likely to work with this particular child; we take care not to say, 'For *that* problem use *this* method' – what we do depends on what our observations tell us of the individual child. However, there are two quite common problems which I think I can suggest particular ways of dealing with: swearing and masturbation. This is because the reinforcers for each of these problems are nearly always the same. Self-injury, which is quite different, is discussed later.

1. *Swearing*

Many people find swearing unpleasant and especially embarrassing in public – which is when it often happens. We may try telling the child not to use such words, that we don't like it, and neither do other people, scold her sharply when she uses the words – and find her swearing goes on unabated. The reinforcement for swearing seems to be, almost always, the attention that it brings (though there may be exceptions to this that I don't know of). So the method worth trying first is extinction. When the swear-words are used, we just don't react. We don't start back, look horrified, tell the child to be quiet, or say anything about it at all. We behave as if we had heard nothing, and continue talking pleasantly of the weather, the neighbour's dog and the price of fish. It is not always easy to do this, especially since, as in other cases where we use extinction, the child is likely to redouble her efforts at first and produce longer, louder and more appalling swear-words. We may have to take friends into our confidence, tell them what we plan to do and ask them to cooperate. If the swearing happens in a really public place we may have to beat a hasty and dignified retreat before the general public's shock becomes reinforcing to the child. If there is one particular public place the child often goes to it can be a good idea to forewarn the people likely to be on the scene. Swearing was one of Ann's problems, as well as disobedience (see page 87), and her mother decided to deal with it using extinction. She went along to the supermarket that she and Ann visited almost every day, talked to the manageress and other staff, and asked them if they too would take no notice of the swearing. Not only did the staff willingly cooperate in this but they would also discreetly tell any potentially horrified customers about what was going on, and ask them to help in the same way. At first Ann's mother made the shopping expeditions at times when the supermarket was likely to be fairly uncrowded, but later, as the swearing became less frequent, she and Ann went at any time.

At the same time of course we may combine extinction with DRO; offer something nice, or tokens to exchange for something bigger, for times when the child does not swear – a token for every half hour or hour, or even half day, when there has been no swearing – and this too may help things along. Ann's mother used both methods, extinction and DRO, as a result of which Ann took to saying 'Oh blow' instead of the things she had said before, and everyone was happy.

2. *Masturbation*

Masturbation can be a problem with either boys or girls though it often seems more intense, more embarrassing and more difficult to control in boys, especially during adolescence. It is especially embarrassing when done in public. In addition, children who masturbate may be unwilling to do anything else, and masturbation may seriously interfere with learning other useful things. So it must be controlled, although we will not want to stop it altogether – after all it may offer the only form of sexual pleasure the child will experience.

Once again, you can be pretty sure what the reinforcer is. But in this case the reinforcer lies within the activity itself – the pleasure the children get from masturbating. So we cannot ensure that they do not get this reinforcement but we may be able to ensure that they only masturbate at certain times, and only in private. We make it clear that they may not masturbate in the streets or the shops or the classroom or the living-room, but may when they are alone and private in their bedrooms. If they understand speech well it may be enough to tell them this and to remind them. If they do not understand speech then it may help to put them in special clothing, like high-sided dungarees, which make it less likely that hands will be slipped into trousers. One boy was also given a cricketer's box to wear which prevented accidental contact with and rubbing of his penis, and this also helped to lessen his urge to masturbate and allowed him to concentrate more easily on other things. These measures will not teach the children not to masturbate (which is not really the aim), and usually the minute the clothing is removed they will return to masturbating; but at least it may be controlled so that it doesn't interfere too much with the rest of their lives, or cause too much embarrassment to those around them.

3. Self-injury

Lastly, a problem that is quite different from the other two in that there is no straightforward way of tackling it: self-injury. There are a number of children who hurt themselves, not accidentally but deliberately; and in some cases sufficiently severely to cause bruises or open wounds, occasionally even endangering their lives, so that, for their own protection, some children have spent their days and nights spread-eagled on a bed, hands and feet tied to the four corners.

Why some children deliberately damage themselves – by banging their heads, poking at their eyes, slapping, pinching, scratching or biting themselves – is uncertain. Many theories have been put forward: some people have thought that children injure themselves because they feel unloved, others that they do it to gain attention; with some children it has seemed that they were more likely to do it if they were unoccupied, others when they were over-excited; some children, it has been suggested, may injure themselves because they actually enjoy the sensation it gives them.

All these ideas have been put to the test in attempts to treat self-injuring children. All have had some success – except the first: if children are given extra love and attention when they injure themselves their rate of self-injury increases (as you might expect from what you know of reinforcement); extra love and attention given when they are not self-injuring does not have this effect but neither does it, by itself, usually result in a lessening of the self-injury.

It seems that the reinforcers for self-injury (what keeps the behaviour going), may be quite different for different children. Furthermore, it may occur for different reasons at different times, or that different forms of self-injury (self-hitting and eye-poking, for example) may have different reinforcers or different causes. All this, added to the specially frightening nature of the behaviour, means that self-injury is a special case. It is one to which there is no simple answer, and one where to attempt a simple remedy may do more harm than good. A book like this one is not the right place to look to for help. It is time to call in the professionals. Your doctor, or the head teacher of your child's school, may be able to advise you on where to go for help. The community team for people with learning disabilities, contacted through the local office of the Department of Social Services, will work with you to devise a way of dealing with the self-injury that will help your child and you.

There is one small exception to this. If the child has only just begun to injure herself, and if the form it takes is not serious – light slapping, for example – as a first move, it may be worth studiously ignoring it. With many children, paying attention to them when they injure themselves has the effect of increasing the number of times they do it. So, when the child begins, we would not comment on what she was doing, not watch her, not pull her hands down. We would turn away from her, and only turn back and give her our full attention when she stopped slapping herself, or whatever. And if this resulted, in a few days or so, in a lessening of the number of times she injured herself we would breathe a sigh of relief; if not, we would set about at once making contact with the professionals. But it is worth trying.

The main points

1. A child's 'bad' behaviours may need to be decreased because they:
   (a) can reduce her opportunities for learning;
   (b) can disturb the lives of people around her.

2. As a first step we try to understand the meaning of the behaviour to the child.

3. We can try to change these behaviours by rearranging the surroundings so as to make the behaviour less likely to occur.

4. DRO – Differential Reinforcement of Other kinds of be-

haviour – involves building up (reinforcing) new, good, behaviours in place of the 'bad' ones.

5. Extinction is a method whereby the reinforcer that has customarily followed the behaviour no longer does so, which should result in the behaviour dying out (being extinguished).

6. At the beginning of an extinction programme we can expect the behaviour to increase (to get worse, if the behaviour is a bad one).

7. Once a behaviour has begun to be treated by extinction it should *never* be reinforced.

8. Extinction can affect (decrease) both bad and good behaviours.

9. Time-out from positive reinforcement involves reinforcement which is continuously available to the child until the bad behaviour occurs, when it disappears for a short time.

10. Brief restraint may be used to interrupt a child's overactive behaviour and to teach her calmer behaviours.

Some practice problems

*1. Think of any public figure you don't care for (TV or pop star, politician, sporting personality, etc.). How would you use:
    (*a*) extinction;
    (*b*) time-out to eliminate one or more of this person's bad behaviours?

*2. Which of the methods discussed – time-out, extinction, restraint, DRO or changing the surroundings – might you use for the following:
    (*a*) A neighbour who often calls with a gift of fruit or flowers from her garden and then stays to tell you about her illnesses over the last twenty years;

(*b*) Your teenage sons who, in spite of being asked politely not to do so, always leave their clothes on the bedroom floor;

(*c*) Your three-year-old who, when you are out shopping, interrupts every conversation you attempt with your friends with demands to be taken to the lavatory;

(*d*) Your ageing mother who asks at the end of every meal she has cooked for you: 'Well, did you enjoy that?';

(*e*) Your elderly cat who has taken to stealing butter?

Are there any of these for which none of these methods would be appropriate? What else would you do? Would you just put up with it?

Part 2: Some Things to Teach

Where Part 1 is concerned with the general principles of behavioural methods, with ways of teaching and of dealing with difficult behaviour, in Part 2 I shall be looking more closely at some particular things that children need to learn, and of particular ways in which we can help them to do so.

There may be people who, eager to get on with the job of teaching their children, skip the first part of this book and turn straight away to the second part. If you do so you may find that some of the words and terms in Part 2 are unfamiliar and that the teaching methods are not explained. All this is dealt with in Part 1. So if Part 2 on its own seems difficult, you could go back and have a look through Part 1.

8. Dressing and Undressing

For the child with learning disabilities, clothes to be put on in the morning and taken off again in the evening (to say nothing of all the shoes, trainers, gumboots, cardigans, jackets and coats that have to be donned and doffed during the day) are just a few more hurdles in a life already full of difficulties and frustrations. Many children master these tasks quite easily but for some children their parents feel that they are so complex as to be hardly worth attempting. Dressing, too, takes place in the morning when time tends to be short: 'We're always in a hurry and he's got to be on that coach so it's easier to dress him myself.' Nevertheless if the child *can* learn to dress herself it will ease the morning rush for her parents, while she herself will have the satisfaction of having mastered another interesting skill.

To teach dressing we use the methods already discussed – reinforcement: prompting and fading: and breaking down the task into small steps (see chapters 3–5). This last seems particularly important. We are so accustomed to putting on our clothes, and put them on so automatically, that it is difficult to realize what a complicated process it is. It is quite an eye-opener to try to analyse exactly what we do, and how we do it, when we (for instance) put on a sock. For a child with learning disabilities such a task may be too much to tackle all at one go; if she tries it she may fail. But if we break down the task into small steps she can cope with learning just one step; then she can learn the next step; and so on, until finally she manages to do the whole task. In this way, learning only a very small part at a time, a child can master tasks which before seemed completely beyond her.

Backward chaining (pages 67–8) also figures largely, because it seems a satisfactory way of teaching dressing: but if forward chaining (breaking the sequence down into small steps, teaching the first step first, then teaching the second step and joining – chaining – it to the first, and so on) appeals to you more for any reason, go ahead and use it. (To do this you could usually reverse the backward chaining scales given.)

Looking at the problem

Before we begin to teach a child to dress herself it is often helpful to get clear in our minds exactly how much she can and can't do for herself. Jack, who was mentioned on page 64, was taught to dress himself after years of being encouraged, cajoled, chivvied, prompted, helped and downright dressed. When his teacher decided to set about teaching him systematically to dress himself, she was not really sure how much of this jumbled process Jack did on his own, and how much, in the event, was done for him. So for four mornings when he dressed she watched carefully to see how much he could do by himself, and how much help he really needed. She noted how many garments he could put on without help and whether it made any difference if his clothes were arranged on his bed in the right order, or if they were then handed to him one at a time. At the end of the four days his teacher found that Jack had never succeeded in putting on his socks; he had managed his vest, pants and shoes once each, his cardigan twice and trousers three times, while his greatest success was with his shirt which he had managed to put on ten times, although he could not button it up. Out of 128 opportunities to put on garments Jack had been successful 18 times; he had managed to put on garments only when they were handed to him in the right order. By now his teacher had a much clearer idea of what Jack was able to do, and of how to set about teaching him.

In the same way we can look at how much a child is able to do in undressing herself. We take her to her room, or the bathroom, or wherever she normally gets undressed, and say,

'Get undressed Carol', and see how much she can do without any help at all. We look at:

1. What garments she can manage – vest, pants, socks, tights, shoes, jumper, cardigan, T-shirt, shirt or blouse, skirt, dress, trousers.
2. Whether she can undo fastenings – buttons, zips, laces, buckles, poppers, Velcro.
3. Whether she hangs up the clothes she takes off, puts them on a chair, or drops them on the floor.

It is usually helpful to set a limit on how long the child will be left to struggle on her own, depending either on time or on the child's behaviour. For example, when we tell Carol to get undressed we might decide to let her try to get out of her sweater for between thirty seconds and a minute, or until she clearly gives up. We would then remove the sweater for her and then let her try on her own with the next garment.

One minor variation of this preliminary analysis of what the child can and cannot do is to try the effect of incentives. Philip (see page 87) never undressed himself at home, although his parents had heard that he did so at his nursery school. After they had attended a course in behavioural methods his parents offered Philip a jelly-tot for every garment he removed without help: within a short space of time Philip became, unaided, stark naked. In this case he did not need to be taught the skills to undress himself but he did need the motivation to use the skills he in fact already possessed.

Teaching dressing

A. *Putting on pants – backward chaining scale*

Suppose it is decided that Bobby should begin to learn to put on his pants. His teacher sits him down, on a chair or on the floor, wherever he is most comfortable: she puts his feet through each of the leg openings of his pants, pulls them up to his knees (or thereabouts), stands Bobby up, and pulls the pants up to about three inches below his waist. Then she guides his hands to the waistband, holds them on to it, says, 'Pull your pants up Bobby', and prompts him to pull them up to his waist. Then she reinforces him.

Bobby can of course be taught to do this step in pulling up his pants not only when he is being dressed in the morning but also every time he goes to the toilet. As he begins to do some of the action himself his teacher fades her prompts, until Bobby is able to pull his pants up the last three inches by himself. Next his teacher pulls up his pants to about three inches lower still – about six inches from his waist – and again Bobby is prompted as much as he needs to be to pull them up. After this the sequence may go as follows (the whole sequence is given for convenience):

Done by adult	*Done by child*
1. Pants pulled up to mid-hips	1. Pulls up to waist
2. Pants pulled up to lower hips	2. Pulls up to waist
3. Pants pulled up to mid-thigh (between thigh and knee)	3. Pulls up to waist
4. Pants pulled up to knees	4. Pulls up to waist
5. Pants pulled up to mid-calf	5. Pulls up to waist
6. Pants put on over both feet to ankles	6. Pulls up to waist
7. One of child's feet put into leg opening	7. Holds waistband, puts other foot in leg opening, pulls pants to waist
8. Pants held spread out in front of child's toes	8. Holds waistband, puts in first one then other foot, pulls pants to waist
9. Pants handed to child right way round	9. Puts on pants and pulls them up
*10. Pants handed to child any way round	10. Gets pants the right way round, puts them on and pulls them up

11. Pants laid out on bed or chair	11. Takes pants, puts them on and pulls them up

* Step 10 may require special teaching – see 'Back-to-front and inside-out', pages 116–17.

How much to teach?

How far the programme goes depends on the child's age, and how well she gets on. With a young or very disabled child we might think it enough, for the time being anyway, to stop at step 9, and reckon that she was doing a good job if she could put on her pants when they were handed to her the right way round. On the other hand with a more capable child we might want to go beyond step 11, and teach the child to take her own pants from the wardrobe or drawer, pick out the right ones to put on, and so on. If our eventual aim is that the child should be able to dress herself entirely without help we must make sure that our training goes far enough for her to be able to do so. When Simon learnt to do up buttons (see page 75) his delighted teacher told her colleagues that he was able now to button up his shirt without any help from her. However, when she arranged for Simon to demonstrate his newly learnt skill her colleagues found that, although Simon could success-fully manipulate the buttons through the buttonholes, he waited before each one for his teacher to start him off by wagging her finger at him and saying 'one', 'two', and so on. So then she had to fade out these prompts until Simon would do up all his buttons on being told, 'Do your buttons up'. Eventually he should learn to do them up without any instruc-tion at all, as a natural consequence of putting on his shirt in the morning.

Putting on trousers can be taught in much the same way as putting on pants. Although they are larger and more compli-cated than pants, some children find trousers easier because there is less chance of getting two feet into one leg-opening. Some children, however, find trousers more difficult because when they are expected to put a foot into the trouser leg they try to shove the foot in flat, without pointing their toes to the ground, so the foot gets stuck in the trouser leg. In this case it may help to have 3 extra steps, between 6 and 7, like this:

Done by adult	*Done by child*
6(*a*) Trousers put on over both feet to ankles	6(*a*) Pulls up to waist
6(*b*) One of child's feet put into trouser leg to ankle, other foot put two-thirds of the way in, with foot pointing to floor	6(*b*) Pushes second foot all the way through, pulls up from ankles to waist
6(*c*) As 6(*b*), but second foot put half-way in, pointing to floor	6(*c*) Pushes second foot through, pulls to waist
6(*d*) As 6(*b*) but second foot put quarter way in, pointing to floor	6(*d*) Pushes second foot through, pulls to waist

During steps 6(*b*), 6(*c*) and 6(*d*) the adult will at first prompt the child to point her foot down the trouser leg, and will gradually fade this prompt so that the child learns to do it for herself. If necessary the same process is carried out with the second foot between steps 7 and 8.

Again, if the trousers don't have an elastic waistband, but an opening at the waist with zip and button it seems best to treat putting on the trousers and doing them up as two separate tasks to be taught separately (see section on 'Fastenings', pages 123–7).

Other garments can be taught in much the same way. At the end of the chapter (pages 120–22) you will find examples of backward chaining scales for teaching putting on different garments, to go over the head (vest/jumper/T-shirt/dress) or round the back (shirt/cardigan/jacket/coat), for socks and for fastenings. (See also 'Making your own adaptations of the scales', pages 114–16.)

Note: I recommend that you do not try to read through all the backward chaining scales as literature: only read them if you want to use them, or read one or two to see how they work. They *do* work, but they are mind-boggling to read cold.

Teaching undressing

Undressing is usually easier for children than dressing, and some children undress enthusiastically all day long. Nevertheless, if a child can't undress herself it may be worth taking the trouble to teach her how to do it. The steps in a backward chaining scale to teach taking off a jumper might be as follows:

B. *Taking off jumper/dress/vest/T-shirt*

Done by adult	*Done by child*
1. Removes jumper completely, leaving child holding it	1. Puts jumper on to chair
2. Pulls jumper up over child's head, takes one arm out of sleeve	2. Grasps other sleeve and pulls off, puts jumper on chair
3. Pulls jumper over child's head, leaving both arms in sleeves	3. Grasps one sleeve and pulls off, then the other and completes
4. Pulls jumper up to and just over child's shoulders	*4. Pulls jumper over head and completes
5. Pulls jumper up to just below child's shoulders	*5. Pulls jumper over head from shoulders and completes
6. Pulls jumper up to rib level	*6. Pulls jumper over head from rib level and completes
	*7. Pulls jumper over head from waist level and completes

* Steps 4 to 7 may be done by the child in one of two ways: either the child crosses her arms in front of her and grasps the right side of the jumper with her left hand and the left side of the jumper with her right hand to pull the jumper over her head; or she puts her arms straight back over her shoulders and grasps the jumper at about shoulder level to pull it off. For some reason women seem to favour the first, and men the second method.

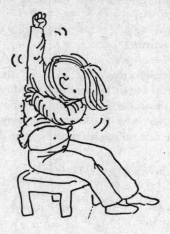

On the whole undressing involves fewer steps than dressing, probably because garments fall off us more easily than they fall on to us. For this reason I have not given backward chaining scales for taking off other garments – they are fairly easy to devise yourself if you want them.

Making your own adaptations of the scales

The backward chaining scales given here are intended only as a guide, and are not meant to be taken as a sacred text. You may find that some different way of putting on a garment suits your child, or you, better than the one given; you can then work out and teach the steps that make up the method you have chosen. For example, some people do not take a jumper off in the way I have described on page 113, first pulling it over the head and then taking the arms out; they prefer to take their arms out first and then pull it over their heads. If this is how you would prefer to do it, it should be fairly easy to adapt the scale. Again, you may find you need extra steps in a scale; to go back to taking off a jumper, the scale on page 113 assumes that the child can learn to pull the jumper over her head all in one step (3 to 4 on this scale). If she finds this very difficult we could insert extra steps: getting the jumper almost but not quite over her head, then getting it half-way over, then pulling it up to her ears, before expecting her to move on to step 4 and pull it right over her head.

You may find, too, that different kinds of garments require slightly different methods. For example, although vest, T-shirt, jumper and dress have been grouped as garments that go over the head, they are not quite the same – vests don't usually have sleeves, for one thing. Again, the crucial step of finding the second armhole may be more difficult with a soft floppy cardigan than it is with a firm jacket. Whenever a particular difficulty arises, the important thing is to work out exactly what the difficulty is; once you have done that it is usually easier to see how it can be got over.

For example, Jack had a particular difficulty at step 2 in learning to put on his sock (see page 122). He managed step 1, pulling up the socks from his ankle, quite easily, but when his teacher moved on to step 2 Jack pulled and tugged at his sock without being able to get it over his heel. His teacher saw that the problem lay in the position in which Jack sat to put on his socks. He would sit on his bed, cross one leg over the other, resting the heel of the crossed-over leg on the other knee and attempt to pull up the sock on that foot. When he had to pull the sock up over the heel it was virtually impossible to get the sock past the barrier formed by his heel resting heavily on his knee, and Jack got very frustrated. His teacher tried to make him keep his foot on the floor and bend down to put the sock on, but Jack refused to do this, and in fact was rather too stout to do so comfortably. In the end his teacher brought in a small chair, and made Jack put his sockless foot on it. She then put the sock over his toe and up to his heel, and by resting his toe on the chair Jack could pull the sock up over his heel. When he moved on to step 5, when the sock was put only over his toes, he first rested his heel on the chair, pulled the sock up to his heel, then rocked his foot to rest his toes on the chair and pulled the sock all the way up.

Again, with some children we find that, with garments like pants, the child successfully achieves the first step – pulling them up to her waist – but manages to pull them up either at the front or at the back, but not both; so that somewhere there is a sagging gap. (The same sort of thing can happen with pulling down jumpers or vests.) So we may have to insert an extra step here, and make sure that the child learns to get the garment pulled straight at front *and* back.

Back-to-front and inside-out

If a child is going to learn to dress herself properly without help she will have to learn to put her clothes on the right way round. To help her learn which is the front and which the back part of her garments it is a good idea to sew a label, or a clearly sewn thread mark, into the back of jumpers, vests, pants, trousers without a front opening, T-shirts and dresses. The child can then be taught to begin putting on the garment by placing it on her bed or chair front side down and with the label uppermost: when she picks it up to put it on, it is facing the same way as she is. Socks seem to be more easily managed if the mark is put on the front.

Which shoe should go on which foot can cause difficulty. Philip (see page 87) would go on and on asking his mother whether he had got them right, even after he was told he had. So his mother made a template for him: she put his shoes down on a piece of cardboard, side by side and slightly apart, and drew round them with a red felt tip. Philip was delighted with this, and kept the template in his bedroom with his shoes resting on it. When he wanted to put on his shoes he went up to them as they stood with their heels towards him on the template, and, standing behind them, put each one on the corresponding foot. He no longer had to ask whether they were right.

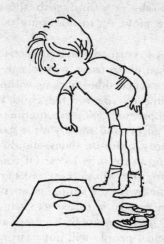

Which is the outside of the garment and which the inside can be taught by showing the child the seams on the inside, and rubbing her thumb along them. If the seams are not obvious, as for instance with socks, or on a garment with raised seams on the outside, again a label on the inside may help. In this case the label on the back of, say, a jumper may be enough but if the child still has difficulty it may be better to sew another label right inside, perhaps on the shoulder. Then the child can be encouraged always to make sure that the garment has the label, or the seams, inside before she starts to put it on.

Organizing the teaching

When we begin teaching a child to dress or undress it is much easier if the clothes are loose, easy to get on and off – especially around the neck; there is something alarming as well as frustrating about having your head stuck half-way inside a constricting woolly tube. (You will see that this is another instance of the use of structural prompts, in that we alter the things the child has to deal with to make it possible for her to learn to cope with them.) Once she is skilful with these easy garments she may be able to move on to managing more sophisticated ones.

At first then we use garments that are constructed as simply as possible – tracksuits, trousers with elasticated waistbands, slip-on or Velcro-fastened shoes, jackets without buttons at the cuffs. All these simplify life for the child learning to dress herself and for the parents. People sometimes ask, why try to teach the child to go beyond these simple garments: why, for instance, when there are slip-on shoes, should the child have to bother with learning to tie shoe-laces? Of course, she needn't, and for those children for whom these tasks are very difficult it may be better to stick with the simple garments. But if she has the ability to learn to deal with extras such as buttons, laces and straps more garments will become available for her to choose from – most people will not want to wear tracksuits all the time. So if she can learn to manage well-fitting clothes and at least some fastenings it may be worth teaching her to do so.

We like to teach activities to a child at the time of day at which those activities normally take place. But many people find early mornings, the normal time for dressing, a rush without adding extra things to be done; it may take too much of the available time to teach a child the rather slow process of dressing herself. In that case we may keep the lessons for the weekend; or we may decide that if we can't teach all the garments together we can at least teach them one at a time – we teach the child to put on her pants, for instance, and dress her in all her other garments ourselves. Then when she has mastered pants and can quickly put them on herself we go on to teach her to put on her vest, and so on. She will learn more slowly, but she will learn.

Finally, don't forget the reinforcement.

The main points

1. To teach dressing, we use prompting, fading, breaking down the activity into small steps, backward chaining, and reinforcement.

2. Forward chaining can be used if preferred.

3. Before starting to teach a child to dress we look to see just how much she can do already and how much she needs to learn.

4. Examples of some backward chaining scales are given. These may be altered or adapted as required.

5. Where problems arise it helps to see how to overcome them if we work out exactly what the difficulty is.

6. Teaching a child to know the back and front of garments is made easier by sewing a label in the back.

7. Teaching the inside and outside of garments can be done by showing the child the seams, or a label, on the inside.

8. We begin teaching dressing with loose, easy, simply constructed garments.

9. If a child can learn to cope with buttons, laces, etc., she will be able to wear a wider variety of clothing.

10. Lessons in dressing are better carried out occasionally, or on one garment at a time, than not at all.

Some practice problems

*1. What steps would you have in a backward chaining scale to teach putting on:
    (a) mitts;
    (b) a woolly hat;
    (c) Wellington boots?

*2. Children differ in what they find the most difficult step, but which would you *expect* to find the most difficult in teaching:

    (*a*) putting on a jumper;
    (*b*) putting on a shirt;
    (*c*) tying a bow?

*3. Can you think of any garment which it might be harder to teach a child to take off than to put on?

Backward chaining scales

A. *Putting on pants, trousers:* pages 109–12
B. *Taking off jumper/dress/vest/T-shirt:* page 113
C. *Putting on vest/jumper/dress/T-shirt*

Done by adult	*Done by child*
1. Vest put over child's head, arms pulled through armholes, vest pulled down to rib level	1. Pulls vest all the way down
2. Vest put over child's head, one arm pulled right through armhole, second arm put half-way through armhole	2. Pushes second arm right through armhole, pulls vest down
3. Vest put over child's head, one arm pulled right through armhole, second hand put to armhole	3. Pushes second arm into and right through armhole, pulls vest down
4. Vest put over child's head, one arm pulled right through armhole, second hand doubled up under vest against ribs	4. Finds armhole with second hand, pushes arm right through and pulls vest down
5. Vest put over child's head, one arm pulled right through	5. Puts second arm into and through armhole, pulls vest down

Done by adult	*Done by child*
6. Vest put over child's head, one arm put half-way through armhole	6. Pushes arm right through armhole, puts second arm through armhole and pulls vest down
7. Vest put over child's head, one hand put to armhole	7. Pushes first arm into and through armhole, puts second arm through armhole and pulls vest down
8. Vest put over child's head, one arm doubled up under vest against ribs	*8. Holds bottom of vest with second hand Finds armhole with first hand, pushes arm right through; puts second arm into and through armhole and pulls vest down
9. Vest put over child's head	9. Puts each arm through armhol and pulls vest down
10. Vest handed to child rolled up and ready to go over head	10. Puts vest over head, puts each arm through armhole and pull: vest down
11. Vest handed to child the right way round	11. Puts vest on
†12. Vest laid out on bed	12. Puts vest on

D. *Putting on shirt/cardigan/jacket/coat*

Done by adult	*Done by child*
1. Both arms put into shirt, one shoulder of shirt pulled up onto child's shoulder	1. Pulls other shoulder of shirt onto own shoulders
2. Both arms put into shirt	2. Pulls shoulders of shirt onto own shoulders
3. One arm put into sleeve, other arm put half in	3. Pushes second arm right in an pulls shirt on

* This part of the step can be included earlier if it would help.
† May require special teaching – see 'Back-to-front and inside-out', p. 116.

Done by adult	Done by child
4. One arm put in sleeve, other arm put to armhole	4. Pushes second arm into arm-hole and through sleeve, pulls shirt on
5. One arm put in sleeve, other arm put near armhole	5. Finds second armhole, pushes arm through and pulls shirt on
6. One arm put in sleeve	6. Finds second armhole, puts arm through and pulls shirt on
7. One arm put partly in	7. Holds shirt by collar, pushes first arm right in, puts second arm in and pulls shirt on
8. Shirt handed in right position, with first armhole in right place	8. Holds shirt by collar, puts first arm in, puts second arm in, pulls shirt on
9. Shirt put on bed/chair in right position (shirt fronts uppermost)	9. Picks up shirt right way and puts on
10. Shirt put out in any position	10. Finds correct sleeve for first arm, puts shirt on

E. Putting on socks (each one in turn)

Done by adult	Done by child
1. Sock put on up to ankle	1. Pulls up sock from ankle
2. Sock put on foot and half over heel	2. Pulls sock over rest of heel and up
3. Sock put on foot just to heel	3. Pulls sock right over heel and up
4. Sock put on to instep	4. Pulls sock from instep and up
5. Sock put over toes	5. Pulls sock up from toes
6. Sock rolled right down to toe and handed to child	6. Puts foot in sock and pulls sock up
7. Sock rolled down to heel and handed to child	7. Puts foot in sock and pulls sock up
8. Sock handed to child	*8. Puts foot in sock right way round and pulls sock up
9. Socks put out on bed or chair	9. Takes socks in turn and puts them on

* May need special teaching – see 'Back-to-front and inside-out', p. 116.

NB: Teaching putting on tights is partly like teaching putting on trousers, partly like teaching putting on socks.

F. *Fastenings*

Tying single knot (on a shoe with black lace on right-hand side and white lace on left-hand side, when toe furthest away from child. Assumes child is right-handed.)

Done by adult	*Done by child*
1. Pick up white lace, lay it diagonally towards toe of shoe: pick up black lace, lay it across white: pick up tips of both laces, pass black behind white and bring tip of black lace under white, bring through	1. Picks up both laces and pulls tight
2. Cross laces as in (1): pick up tips of both laces straight up in air, keep white lace taut, slacken tension on black lace, pass black behind white and leave tip of black just through crossing of laces	2. Pulls black lace through and pulls both laces tight
3. Cross laces as in (1)	3. Picks up tips of both laces straight up in air, keeps white lace taut, slackens tension on black lace, passes black behind and under white, pulls tight
4. Pick up white lace and lay diagonally towards toe of shoe	4. Picks up black lace, lays it across white: picks up tips of both laces straight up in air, keeps white lace taut, slackens tension on black lace, passes black behind and under white, pulls tight

Done by adult	*Done by child*
5. Hands shoe to child	5. Picks up white lace, lays it diagonally towards toe of shoe: picks up black lace, lays it across white: picks up tips of both laces straight up in air, keeps white lace taut, slackens tension on black lace, passes black behind and under white and pulls tight

Tying a bow (on a shoe with one black and one white lace, as above. Assumes single knot already tied.)

1. Pick up white lace in the middle, pinch it together to form loop, pass black lace round white loop, push through and pull out black loop	1. Holds white loop with left hand, black loop with right hand and pulls tight
2. Make loop with white lace, pass black lace round white loop, push black loop just through	2. Pinches looped tip of black lace, pulls through and pulls both loops tight
3. Make loop with white lace, pass black lace round white	3. With first finger of left hand pushes black lace under white loop against right thumb, pulls through and pulls both loops tight
4. Make loop with white lace, give middle of black lace to child	4. Wraps black lace round white loop, pushes through and pulls both loops tight
5. Make loop with white lace	5. Picks up black lace in middle, wraps round white loop, pushes through and pulls both loops tight
6. Gives middle of white lace to child	6. With right hand pinches white lace to form loop, wraps black lace round white loop, pushes through and pulls both loops tight

Done by child

7. With right hand picks up white lace in the middle, makes a loop, wraps round black lace, pushes through and pulls both loops tight

Zips

NB Most zips need to be held and straightened from the bottom, but men usually straighten trouser zips from the top.

Done by adult	*Done by child*
1. Hold bottom (or top) of zip (to straighten it), pull zip all the way up.	1. Turns tag of zip down and presses it flat
2. Pull zip three-quarters up	2. Holds top (or bottom) of zip with one hand, pulls up the last quarter, turns tag down
3. Pull zip half up	3. Holds top/bottom of zip, pulls up last half, turns tag down
4. Pull zip quarter up	4. Holds top/bottom of zip, pulls up last three-quarters, turns tag down
	5. Holds top/bottom of zip, pulls it right up, turns tag down

These steps are suitable for zips that are fixed at the bottom, for instance those in skirts or trousers.

If the zip is one that comes completely apart, as in an anorak, three further steps will be needed. In this case the straightening hand has to be at the bottom of the zip.

5. Seats slide part of zip closure in holder part	
6. Puts slide part of zip closure partly in holder	6. Seats slide part of zip closure fully in holder part and pulls up

Done by adult	*Done by child*
7. Puts slide and holder parts of zip closure side by side	7. Seats slide part of closure in holder part and pulls up
	8. Closes bottom of zip and pulls up

Buttons

It is best to start with large buttons and fairly loose button-holes, as for instance on pyjamas. This is better than teaching buttoning on a special button frame, or on a garment that is laid out in front of the child, as this is rather different from buttoning garments on her own body. Later the child can learn to do up smaller buttons.

The instructions given are for a girl; for boys, reverse the indications for left and right hand.

Done by adult	*Done by child*
1. Push button three-quarters through the buttonhole	1. Holds edge of buttonhole band in left hand, side of button in right, pulls button through
2. Push button half through buttonhole	2. Holds buttonhole band and button as above, pulls button through
3. Push button quarter way through buttonhole	3. Holds buttonhole band with left hand, pushes button with thumb of that hand, holds button with right hand and pulls through
4. Put edge of button to buttonhole	4. Holds button with left hand, buttonhole band with right hand hear buttonhole: pushes button half-way through, transfers button to right hand, band to left hand, and pulls through
5. Put button opposite appropriate buttonhole	5. Inserts edge of button into buttonhole with left hand, transfers to right and pulls through

Done by child

6. Feels upwards from the bottom to find the button and buttonhole opposite each other and does up the button

9. Washing

To teach a child to wash herself we use prompting, fading and, as always, reinforcement. Very important, too, are backward chaining and breaking down each activity into small steps. So for each one I have given a backward chaining scale; as before (page 114) you should take these only as rough guides, and should make your own adaptations of them where you want to, or where you think some other method would suit you, or your child, better than the one given.

Teaching a child to wash herself can include teaching her to:

wash her hands
wash her face
clean her nails
dry her hands and face
clean her teeth
bath herself
dry herself after a bath
wash her hair
know when she needs to wash.

Washing hands

For a child to wash her hands by herself she must be able to:

1. Go to the basin
2. Put in the plug
3. Turn on the cold tap
4. Turn on the hot tap
5. When sufficient water in the basin turn off the hot tap
6. Turn off the cold tap

7. Take the soap
8. Put hands and soap in the water
9. Take soap and hands out of the water, rub soap between hands
10. Put soap down
11. Rub palms and fingers together
12. Rub hands together, interlacing fingers
13. Rub palm and fingers of right hand over back and fingers of left hand
14. Rub palm and fingers of left hand over back and fingers of right hand
15. Rinse hands in water
16. Pull out plug.

We can teach the child to wash her hands by prompting her right through the process, fading our prompts first on step 16, and reinforcing her for completing the washing. When she is able to pull out the plug by herself we begin fading the prompts on rinsing, and so on.

Sometimes children get quite skilful at some earlier parts of the process – for example, turning on the taps – before they have mastered later steps such as turning them off or taking the soap. There seems no point in insisting on prompts where they are not necessary – we let the child do as much and as independently as she can. But we would continue concentrating our teaching at the end of the scale, with the main reinforcement at the end (there is nothing to stop us giving squeals of delight at anything the child can do along the way).

Washing face

Faces can be washed with or without soap, with or without a cloth. How we teach the child to wash her face depends on what sort of a face-wash we are after but probably the easiest way is to teach a child to wash her face with a cloth and without soap. The sequence might be:

1. Go to the basin
2. Take her face-cloth
3. Turn on tap
4. Wet face-cloth
5. Turn off tap
6. Bend over basin
7. Rub cloth all over face
8. Turn on tap
9. Rinse cloth
10. Turn off tap
11. Squeeze out cloth
12. Put cloth away.

It will help her to find her own face-cloth if it is quite different from everyone else's. If she is washing her face at the same time as her hands she can miss out steps 1, 3, 5, 8 and 10.

Cleaning nails

This is fairly advanced (and some of us may feel, judging by the fingernails of our children, that we aren't very good at teaching it). However, it can be taught. The sequence for a child who has already got a basinful of water for washing her hands could be:

1. Pick up nailbrush
2. Wet nailbrush in water
3. Rub nailbrush on soap
4. Brush fingernails of left hand
5. Brush thumbnail of left hand
6. Rinse nailbrush in water
7. Rub nailbrush on soap
8. Brush fingernails of right hand
9. Brush thumbnail of right hand
10. Rinse nailbrush

11. Put nailbrush down
12. Rinse hands.

A fairly soft, unspiky nailbrush will help prevent her from being frightened of being hurt. She will also have to be encouraged to continue the brushing (steps 4, 5, 8 and 9) until her nails are clean: it may be worth having a little extra reinforcement for the completion of each of these steps and deliberately withholding it until all the dirt has gone.

Drying hands and face

The child should:

1. Take her towel
2. Hold it in one hand and rub the towel over the palm and back of the other
3. Hold the towel in the other hand and rub it over the palm and back of the first
4. Rub the towel all over her face
5. Put the towel back.

The main problem here is to make sure that she dries her hands and face thoroughly. This might be dealt with by having extra reinforcement for these steps and not giving it until she is really dry, as with the fingernails.

Cleaning teeth

This is one of the most important of the washing tasks, one of the most difficult to teach, and probably the one which it is most difficult to ensure has been done properly. Again, a not-too-tough brush is advisable (get your dentist's advice on this, as well as on the best size and shape of toothbrush to use) plus a toothpaste the child likes.

Then the steps might be:

1. Takes the toothpaste
2. Unscrews the cap from the toothpaste
3. Puts the cap down
4. Takes her own toothbrush
5. Squeezes out half an inch of toothpaste onto the tooth-brush
6. Puts toothbrush down
7. Puts cap back on toothpaste
8. Takes toothbrush
9. Brushes downwards on outer surfaces of all upper teeth
10. Brushes upwards on outer surfaces of all lower teeth
11. Brushes downwards on inner surfaces of all upper teeth
12. Brushes upwards on inner surfaces of all lower teeth
13. Brushes to and fro on biting surfaces of upper and lower teeth
14. Puts down brush
15. Takes tooth-mug
16. Turns on tap
17. Fills mug with water
18. Turns off tap
19. Rinses mouth and spits out three times
20. Rinses toothbrush
21. Puts toothbrush away
22. Wipes mouth on towel.

The particular difficulty here is likely to be brushing the inner surfaces of the teeth, which is awkward. If steps 9, 10, 11 and 12 are too big and the child has difficulty in learning them, each one could be broken down into three – brushes front, brushes left side, brushes right side.

Many dentists recommend that all children should use electric toothbrushes, as they do a better job of tooth cleaning and gum massage than do the children or their parents. Children often like the sensation of having the electric toothbrush in their mouth, and in this case it is easy to switch to using one. Some children, though, do not like it or are frightened by it, and then it may be worth trying *graded practice* (see page

181). We would have the electric toothbrush lying around in
the bathroom while the child was washing or having her teeth
cleaned with an ordinary brush; occasionally we would try to
get her to put the brush (not switched on) in her mouth. Then,
with it still well away from the child, we would switch it on
and leave it running; when she seemed quite comfortable with
that we would bring it a little nearer, then a little nearer still;
then we would touch it on our own hand, then lightly on hers,
if necessary with a cloth laid over it at first; then on her arm,
shoulder, neck; then we would invite her to put it, just for a
moment, in her mouth, then for a little longer; then actually to
touch a tooth. You get the idea.

Bathing

This again is a complicated activity, and most children do not
as a rule bath themselves completely independently until they
are about 8 or 9. The whole process includes running the bath
and getting the temperature right, washing in the bath, getting
out, letting out the bath water, drying all over and putting on
pyjamas or other clothes.

Since scalding water is extremely dangerous we should continue to supervise the running of the bath until we are quite
sure that the child can test the temperature safely. Washing
and drying are taught in much the same way as washing hands
and face, except that a wider area is covered and the washing
may be done with a cloth.

Some children develop fears of bathing, and refuses to get
into a bath. This happened with Simon (pages 75 and 111): he
had no baths at all between the ages of five and eleven. Here
again his teacher used graded practice (see page 181). At first she
encouraged him to play with favourite toys in the bathroom,
gradually moving them nearer and nearer the bath: then she
put some toys on the edge and later into the (empty) bath, so
that Simon had to lean over the edge of the bath to play with
them. When Simon was quite happy about this she popped

him into the bath to play, and later began taking off some of his clothes while he sat in the bath. When Simon was happy to play in the bath with no clothes on she ran a few drops of water into the bath, and when this became more than just a few drops she put in some bubble bath that Simon enjoyed playing with. Gradually the bath was made deeper and the water was gently stroked over Simon's legs, his arms, his back, his front and finally his neck and face. Simon now baths regularly like anyone else.

Hair washing

This is most easily taught in the bath. Since shampoos are mostly made of detergent it is best if the child washes her hair first with the shampoo, rinses it, and then washes the rest of herself with soap afterwards. The sequence might be:

1. Wets her hair in the bath (either by dipping her head in the bath or by pouring bath water over it);
2. Unscrews the cap of the shampoo bottle;
3. Pours a little shampoo in her hand;
4. Puts down the shampoo bottle;
5. Rubs the shampoo into a lather all over her hair;
6. Rinses her hair by wetting it as in (1) above.

The most common difficulty is that the child may be scared of having water run down over her face and getting soap in her eyes. A non-stinging shampoo, and a shampoo shield to hold the water back from her face (see Appendix 4, 'Aids and Equipment') may help.

After she has washed her hair, the child should be taught to dry it with a towel, or, with careful supervision, an electric hair dryer.

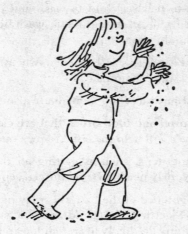

Knowing when a wash is needed

Most children can get used to the routine of a regular bath. Once they have learnt to wash their hands it should not be too difficult to teach them to wash them before meals and after going to the toilet. It may be rather more difficult to teach a child to recognize and deal with dirty hands or face in between times – when she is going shopping or to visit friends, or if she comes indoors very, very dirty. If she does not seem to notice that she needs a wash we might ask, 'Do you want a wash?', prompt her to look at her hands, and if necessary point out the dirt on them. Later the question and the prompt might be gradually faded (see page 65) until eventually she is able to see for herself when her hands are dirty and need a wash.

The main points

1. We may want to teach a child to wash and dry her hands and face, clean her nails, clean her teeth, wash her hair, and to know when she should wash.

2. In each case the process is broken down into small steps and taught by backward chaining.

3. Prompting, fading and reinforcement are also used.

4. A face-cloth, towel and toothbrush that are clearly different from everyone else's will help the child to pick out her own.

5. Some important steps, such as getting all the dirt off, or drying thoroughly, may need to be reinforced separately.

6. If a child is frightened of the bath this may be tackled using graded practice — getting the child from a situation quite different from bathing gradually nearer and nearer real bathing, making sure that she is always happy and relaxed.

Some practice problems

*1. How would you set about teaching Bobby to get the bathwater temperature right?

*2. How dirty is dirty? Or, how do *you* decide your hands need washing?

10. Dry Pants, Dry Bed

Toilet training is an important part of all children's early learning, and even modern parents, who are not too fussed about early training, are usually pleased to see an end to nappies and the washing of knickers. Some children may become trained as young as one year old but for many it is a much longer process: in one large study only just over half of the non-disabled 4-year-olds were reliably toilet-trained.* So it is not surprising if it seems rather a slow business for children with learning disabilities.

Training

Most children become toilet trained through a combination of imitation, parental pleasure and displeasure, and luck. When a child is not making progress in the normal way something more systematic must be tried. The methods we use are likely to rely mainly on reinforcement of the proper use of the toilet and withholding reinforcement from wetting and soiling in places other than the toilet.

With even quite small babies some mothers become very skilful at knowing when their babies are likely to wet or soil, and are able to 'catch' them on the pot. They often say that it is not the babies who are trained but they themselves, and this is probably right. Nevertheless a mother who can 'catch' her child in this way has a lot going for her; the child can be reinforced for performing on the pot, even if it is the mother's effort and not the child's that has brought this about. If she is

* J. & E. Newson, *Four Years Old in an Urban Community*, London, George Allen & Unwin, 1968; Penguin Books, 1970.

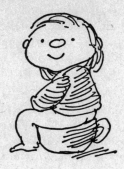

consistently reinforced for performing on the pot she will,
when she is old enough, gradually come to realize the association between what he does and the reinforcement, and become
more ready to perform of her own accord. So 'catching' and
reinforcing are good ways to begin training. With an older
child we can often do much the same; observing her carefully
to see when she is most likely to wet or soil, and putting her on
the toilet at these times.

Some children, however, are not as regular in their habits.
Six-year-old Julie had been so unpredictable that her mother
had given up trying to catch her, and Julie was in nappies
night and day. When her mother decided to make a big effort
to toilet train her she first of all had to take her out of nappies.
She put Julie into trainer pants, made of terry towelling, which
absorbed a good deal if Julie had an accident but, like ordinary
pants, were easy and quick to take off and put on. She decided
she would put Julie on the pot every half hour, and would keep
her there until she performed, or for at least two minutes. In
this way there was a good chance that occasionally Julie would
perform on the pot; when that happened Julie's mother seized
the chance to shower her with reinforcement.

As Julie wasn't keen on staying on the pot for two minutes
her mother stayed beside her, putting her back whenever she
tried to get off. A potty chair can help a child feel safe on the
pot and straps can be fitted to put round the child which will

encourage her to stay on the pot (see Appendix 4, 'Aids and Equipment'). Julie was also given one or two toys or favourite belongings to play with, especially at first, when her mother wanted the whole business of potting to be a pleasant and rewarding one for Julie. Later when Julie had accepted the routine of sitting on the pot her mother began to fade out the toys a bit, to encourage Julie to concentrate on what she was supposed to be doing.

Julie's mother kept a record of how the training went: she recorded for each half hour whether Julie's pants were wet or dry when she was taken to the pot and whether or not she used the pot. If her mother had found that Julie was almost always wet, and that she hardly ever used the pot she might have thought it worth while, for a time at least, putting Julie on the pot every fifteen minutes in the hope of 'catching' her, and of getting the opportunity to reinforce her. Once Julie began to realize that using the pot was followed by reinforcement, and began to use it more often, her mother could gradually space out the times Julie was put on the pot.

All sorts of things may contribute towards the decision to embark on toilet training – what stage the child seems to be at, how much time her mother has to spare just then, ups and downs in the rest of the family, and so on. Everything else being equal many mothers prefer to start in the summer, when the child will be wearing thinner and fewer clothes, so accidents can be spotted more quickly and changing is easier; and puddles and damp clothes seem somehow less important in the summer – Nature is on our side where drying is concerned.

Accidents

During her training Julie naturally had a good many accidents, when she wet or soiled her pants. Her pants then had to be changed, and her mother soon realized that this pants-changing was in many ways a very enjoyable time for Julie. She loved attention, and here she had her mother all to herself for ten minutes or so; in addition her mother used at these times to talk to her a great deal, scolding her, commenting on what was going on, praising her for pulling up her pants, and so on. If Julie was soiled her mother often used to give her a warm bath, as this seemed the quickest way to get her cleaned up, and then Julie would play in the water and enjoy being hugged dry in the towel. Once her mother realized that the whole business of changing pants was a rewarding one for Julie she decided to make it rather different. Now when she was changing her Julie's mother remained neutral, not scolding, not praising, indeed talking very little. When Julie was soiled she was cleaned up with warm water from a basin. However, when she managed to go for a whole day without being soiled her mother gave her an extra-long enjoyable bath and extra towel-hugging in the evening: she did not want Julie to lose this pleasure, only for it to follow her good rather than her less good kinds of behaviour.

Wiping up

A child who is to be completely independent for toileting needs to learn to wipe her bottom after defecating. This is quite an advanced skill, which we probably would not attempt to teach unless the child was physically fairly skilful, and also quite confident and secure on the toilet seat. Then we teach her by physical prompting – putting the toilet paper in her hand, closing our hand round hers and making the necessary movements to wipe her bottom and drop the paper into the toilet. One difficulty is knowing when to stop wiping: so we prompt the child to look at the paper which she has just used, and if it is dirty to take another piece, only stopping when the piece she has just wiped herself with is clean or almost clean.

Girls should be taught to wipe themselves from front to back, as wiping in the opposite direction can cause urinary infections. Boys, for whom it is less important, are apparently likely to wipe from front to back anyway.

'I want to go!'

When a child has learnt to keep herself dry and to use the toilet appropriately it may be helpful to her if she can let people know when she wants to go: if, for instance, she is away from home, or can't open doors, or needs help with her clothes or with getting on and off the toilet. So, right from the early stages of the training, it is a good idea to begin to teach her to use some signal whenever she is taken to the toilet. If she can talk we can when taking her always say 'Toilet' (or any other word normally used); if she does not talk we can use the word plus a 'Toilet' sign; or the word plus any kind of sign the child herself tends to use, such as clutching at the front of her knickers. (Even if this last is a bit unlovely it may be worth using it to teach her to indicate her wants – if she learns it we can later, in the same way, pair it with and teach her a more sophisticated sign.) After a few days of always using the signal when we take her to the toilet we can go on to prompting her to imitate the signal; later still, fade the prompts, and then go on to using a question instead of only modelling the response – 'What do you want? Say, "Toilet"'; or 'What do you want? Do "Toilet"', plus whatever sign she knows or is learning. Later again we fade this too (see page 64) until the child is able to ask for the toilet when she wants it.

Help from the surroundings

Julie's toilet training was begun on a pot, as happens with most small children, and a special potty chair to help her sit more securely, and perhaps a musical potty which plays a tune when she uses it, might help (see Appendix 4, 'Aids and Equipment'). In time, however, she will need to learn to use an ordinary toilet, as part of becoming more grown-up and also to make it easier for her to go to the toilet when she is away from home. Many small children find the big toilet alarming, with its big opening through which a small person might slide. Trainer seats, which fit between the ordinary toilet seat and the bowl and make a smaller seat for the child to sit on, can be a help. These are obtainable from most large chemists. Children often find it difficult to climb up on to the high seat; a firm box that they can climb on to first, and on which they can rest their feet while sitting on the toilet, makes it easier and adds to the child's feeling of security. For a child who is very nervous of sitting on the toilet seat it may be worth fixing a handle to the wall beside the toilet for her to hold on to. Where to keep the toilet paper can be a problem: it must be available for the child to use, but sometimes a child gets the idea that it is hilarious to unwind yards of paper and push it down the toilet. In this case it may be a good idea to put the main roll or packet of paper on a high shelf out of reach of the child and keep a few pieces, to be replaced as necessary, at toilet-seat height for legitimate use.

Intensive programmes

If, in spite of putting into practice the ideas discussed above, a child still makes little progress with toilet training we may have to resort to more drastic methods, along the lines of programmes devised by Drs Nathan Azrin and Robert Foxx in America. These programmes concentrate full-time on toileting, and include very frequent regular checks on pants, extra liquids for the child to drink, frequent trips to the toilet, massive reinforcement for success and mild discouragement for accidents. Lennie was 9 years old and had never been clean and dry, although there seemed no real reason why he should not be. His teacher decided to try an intensive programme with him. First she set up the toilet area with a table, two chairs, some toys, a cup, a bottle of Lennie's favourite orange squash, several spare pairs of pants, a kitchen timer, several bars of Lennie's favourite milk flake chocolate and a record sheet. She planned to carry out Lennie's programme from 9.30 in the morning till 12, when he would go to lunch, and again from 12.30 to 3.30 in the afternoon. Lennie was taken to the toilet area at 9.30, and his teacher felt his pants: for a wonder, they were dry. '*Good boy*, Lennie, you've got *dry pants*!' she said in a tone of voice doubtless used by somebody conveying to Wellington the result of the battle of Waterloo. She put his hand to his pants and made him feel them himself, once again saying, 'Good boy, *dry* pants', and she broke off a little bit of chocolate flake and gave it to him. When he, delightedly, had eaten it she filled the cup with diluted orange squash and gave him as much as he would drink – two cups. The point of these extra fluids is to increase the number of times Lennie will want to pass water, hopefully into the toilet so that he can be reinforced for his success, but even if the result is sometimes wet pants this, too, can be used as part of the teaching process. His teacher waited for about a minute after he had had his drink and then said, 'Go to the toilet, Lennie'. Lennie didn't budge from his chair, so she gently prompted him to go to the toilet, pull down his pants and sit on the toilet. She set the kitchen timer to twenty minutes: Lennie was to sit on the toilet for twenty minutes or until he used it. After a few moments Lennie had had enough of sitting on the toilet and he tried to get off it, but his teacher pushed him back, and pushed him back every time he tried to stand up, until eventually he gave up and just sat there.

Seventeen minutes went by, and then came the welcome sound of splashing. The reaction Lennie got now was like that customarily reserved for the liberator of a beleaguered city – arms flung round him, kisses showered on him, his praises sung to the skies, and a generous wodge of chocolate flake popped in his mouth. Then his teacher allowed him to stand up, she prompted him to pull up his pants, and led him back to the table. For the next five minutes they played with the toys. His teacher then felt, and prompted him to feel, his

Name: Lennie

Date: 6.7.92

Time	9.30	10	10.30	11	11.30	
Fluids given	✓	✓	water	✓	✓	
Amount taken	2 cups	1 cup	⅓ cup	1 cup	1½ cups	
Waited 1 minute	✓	✓	✓	✓	✓	
Child goes to toilet without prompting	—	—	—	—	✓	
Sent to toilet	✓	✓	✓	✓		
Used toilet: Yes	✓	—	✓	✓	✓	
Time taken	17′	—	11′	12′	2′	
Reinf. given	✓	—	✓	✓	✓ + +!	
No		✓				
Five-min. checks	✓✓	✓✓	✓✓✓	✓✓✓	✓✓✓✓	
Dry	✓✓	✓	✓✓✓	✓✓✓	✓✓✓✓	
Chocolate given	✓✓	✓✓	×	✓✓✓	✓✓✓✓	
Wet		✓				
Discouragement given		✓				
Comments	Loves reinforcer	Upset at not getting reinforcer	Sits better	Seems to know what he needs to do to get reinforcer	Triumph	

pants. They were dry, both then and at the following five-minute check, so each time Lennie was praised and given a small piece of chocolate flake. By now it was 10 o'clock and time to start the whole process again. Lennie was again given as much diluted orange squash as he would take – a cupful –

and as before he was prompted to go to the toilet, but this time he didn't use it. At the end of twenty minutes his teacher stood him up without comment, and they returned to the toys. At the next five-minute pants check, Lennie's pants were damp. His teacher made him feel them, shook her head and said sadly and with emphasis, 'That's *bad*, Lennie, your pants are *wet*.' She picked up a piece of chocolate and showed it to him, shook her head again and said, 'No chocolate, your pants are *wet*,' and put the piece down again. Now she helped Lennie to take off his pants, put on a clean pair and rinse his pants out in cold water. (This is the mild discouragement.) She did not praise him for any of this. They then returned to the table, but Lennie's teacher did not play with him or talk to him for the next five minutes but made him sit quietly in the chair. At the next pants check his pants were dry: she praised him, but did not give him any chocolate flake, and, when he was next due for fluids, he had plain water instead of orange squash. (She had decided that when he had wet his pants he should miss out on the foods for a time, to help to impress on him that it was not a good idea to wet his pants. The next time he got the enjoyable food and drinks was after the next time he used the toilet, at about 10.42 a.m. If he had not used the toilet at this time he would have got the chocolate the next time after this that his pants were dry.)

So the morning wore on – rather slowly, it must be admitted, for Lennie's teacher. Her reward, however, was at hand. At 11.30 a.m., after he had had his drink, Lennie took himself, unprompted, to the toilet, and used it after only two minutes. After nine years of incontinence he had cottoned on to the fact that it was worth his while to use the toilet and to keep his pants dry.

Opposite is the record that Lennie's teacher kept of his first morning of the intensive programme.

Maintaining progress

Lennie responded unusually quickly to the intensive toilet training programme – it can take several days for children to reach the stage that he got to in one morning. His teacher kept up the programme for another three days, to make sure that his success was not accidental; Lennie continued using the toilet, having dry pants, and enjoying the reinforcement he was given. Next, his teacher began to fade out the intensive programme: first the table and chairs were put outside the toilet area, then further up the corridor, then into his normal classroom. The pants checks took place now every ten minutes, then every fifteen, then on the half hour. The extra liquids were dropped. Lennie continued to get food reinforcers every time he used the toilet but only now and again for dry pants, though he was always praised. He was always reinforced if he went of his own accord and used the toilet, and now he was only told to go if he had not been for an hour. If he wet his pants, as he did with less and less frequency, he was told that was bad, was helped to change his pants and wash them out, and did not receive the food the next time that that was due.

After two weeks of this 'faded' programme Lennie returned to normal work in his classroom. He went to the toilet at the normal times – before and after meals, and so on – with the other children, and his pants were occasionally checked at these times. Every now and again as well as the praise that all the children got for using the toilet Lennie got a piece of his chocolate flake. Later still even the pants checks and the chocolate were discontinued. Lennie was back to his former routine with the one difference – he was no longer wet, smelly and uncomfortable.

Variations in intensive programmes

Lennie's teacher set up his intensive programme on an all-day basis because she thought this would be the quickest way to get results, and because she was able to do so – she had enough staff working with her who could be with the other children while she was with Lennie. If this had not been possible she might have run the programme in the mornings only, or even just for a couple of hours each day – progress would be likely to be slower but better than if there were no programme at all. Again, if Lennie's teacher had not been able herself to devote the whole day to the programme she might well have enlisted the help of others, to take half-hour shifts; in this case it would be important that everybody was aware of all the details of the programme, and carried it out in exactly the same way as everyone else. The shift system does have the advantage of lessening the tedium for the teacher.

Night-time training

Learning not to wet the bed is harder for most children than learning not to wet their pants, because when they are asleep they have less control over what is going on. However, there are some ideas we can try out to help the child become dry at night.

First, a couple of things that hardly ever help. Punishment is said to be almost always ineffective (and seldom used by parents nowadays), and limiting drinks in the evening makes little difference. Many mothers of bedwetters do try cutting down the amount their children drink in the evening but unless they are drinking a great deal this is unlikely to have much effect.

Now to go on to some ideas that may help.

Medical help

A very few children may have some medical condition which makes it difficult for them not to wet the bed; it is rare, but may be worth checking. Drugs, too, help a small number of children, so it may be worth taking a child to the doctor and asking for advice about bed-wetting.

Potties and night-lights

A child may be put off getting up at night if she has to go out of her room to the toilet; so, if she has not already got one, it may be worth giving her a pot by her bed. Again, she may dislike getting up in the dark, so an electric night-light, or a light left on on the landing, may help. (In our family we only gave up having the landing light on all night when our youngest was sixteen – admittedly it had become a habit and we had forgotten why we left it on.)

Lifting

Many parents lift the child late at night and put her on the pot, and this may help her to go through the night without wetting her bed earlier than she otherwise would have done. If, when she is lifted, she is regularly already wet, it may be worth lifting her progressively earlier in the evening until you find a time when she is regularly dry. She can then be rewarded for being dry at this time. After a week or so you can begin lifting her very slightly later, advancing the time at which she is lifted, by, say, five minutes at a time. The idea is that, although she will still be dry, she will begin to associate the lifting with a gradually more and more full bladder, so that eventually the full bladder itself will wake her.

Star charts

Some children respond well to a star chart with a star to stick on for every dry night. For some, just seeing the star go on to the chart and the praise and attention that go with it seems to be reinforcement enough, but for others it may be more effective if there are exchange reinforcers, so many stars to be exchanged for the reinforcer (see chapter 4).

Pants and bedside alarms

Most children learn, in due course, to wake up when their bladders are full, to get out of bed and go to the toilet. For bedwetters the full bladder is not enough to wake them and they may need to learn to associate the feeling of a full bladder with waking. This is where the toilet training alarms come in. In the pants alarm version the child wears a small noise box fastened (Velcroed) to her pyjama jacket; this is connected to a detector plate which can be fitted in a small 'panty-shield' type of pad or worn between two pairs of pants. (For boys the detector is put between two pairs of pants over the Y-front pouch.) When the child begins to wet, a few drops of liquid (urine) are enough to close an electrical circuit, which sets off the noise box, which wakes the child, who then goes to the toilet. (The apparatus is so constructed that there is no chance of the child getting an electric shock.) As she has passed only a few drops of urine before she is woken she gradually begins to associate the feeling of fullness of her bladder with waking up; in time she no longer needs the alarm.

This way of treating bed-wetting is said to be by far the most effective, and success rates of 60 to 100 per cent have been reported. It does have its complications. If the bed-wetter sleeps in a room with other children the bell may wake them as well, and cause disruption to the family. With most children it is usually not recommended where the child is under seven years old, as she may get in a muddle when she wakes, not go to the toilet properly or not remake the bed adequately after-wards. All this may apply to a child with learning disabilities, too. However, the apparatus can be used slightly differently, for instance by putting the noise box in the parents' room instead of in the child's, so that when it sounds one or other parent wakes and goes quickly to her and lifts and organizes her. If this causes too much disruption of the parents' nights it may be worth while to connect up the apparatus, and make use of it, in the evenings only, when they are awake anyway, switching it off when they themselves go to bed. A lot depends on how desperate they are for the child to stop wetting the bed.

There are several variations on the apparatus available: louder alarms for heavy sleepers, a 'bedside alarm' with a mat to go on the mattress instead of the detector inside the pants and the noise box on a bedside table instead of fixed to the pyjamas, a vibrator to wake the sleeper in place of the noise. An excellent guide to all these systems, including clear instructions on how to use them, is available from ERIC (see Appendix 4) though it also recommends that any programme is undertaken with professional help, from a doctor, psychologist, health visitor or school nurse. Failing this, ERIC runs a telephone helpline service which can be contacted for advice.

The alarms can be borrowed (subject to availability) free of charge from the NHS – ask your doctor, school nurse or enuresis clinic – or bought direct from ERIC.

The main points

1. A good way to start training a child is to see when she is most likely to wet or soil, and 'catch' her on the pot.

2. If the child's habits are not regular enough for this, half-hour toileting can be tried.

3. Trainer pants are easier to manage than nappies.

4. It is probably best to clean a child up neutrally after a toileting accident, especially if she likes attention.

5. The child can be taught to wipe her bottom by prompting her to do it.

6. It is helpful to teach the child to indicate, either by a word or a sign, when she wants to go to the toilet.

7. A potty chair, a toilet seat, a step up to the toilet, a handrail, can all help the child to feel more secure; keeping

most of the toilet paper out of reach avoids having it stuffed down the toilet.

8. An intensive toilet programme includes: full-time concentration on toileting, frequent pants checks, extra fluids, massive reinforcement for success and mild discouragement for accidents.

9. The programme should be gradually faded out.

10. If an intensive programme all day is not possible a partial one is probably better than nothing.

11. Night-time training:

(*a*) punishment and restricting fluids do not usually help much;

(*b*) it is worth asking the child's doctor whether she can help;

(*c*) a potty by the bed, or a night-light, may be useful;

(*d*) it may be worth lifting the child and potting her some time after she has gone to sleep. If a time can be found when the child is dry she can be lifted then; gradually the time at which she is lifted can be advanced;

(*e*) star charts for dry beds work for some children;

(*f*) a pants alarm may help a child to learn not to wet the bed.

Some practice problems

What would you do if the child you were training always wet two minutes after she came off the toilet, even if she had been sitting there for half an hour or so?

11. Eating and Table Manners

Teaching a child to feed herself is often one of our most enjoyable tasks. Most children like their food, so the reinforcer for them is the food itself, and they are usually willing to make an effort to learn this interesting skill. Once again, teaching relies mainly on backward chaining, prompting and fading – this last, fading, seems particularly important in teaching feeding.

A list of aids to teaching feeding, together with the names and addresses of suppliers, can be found in Appendix 4, 'Aids and Equipment.'

Sitting in a good position

Before starting to teach a child to feed herself we make sure she is sitting in a good position. She should be sitting securely in the chair, supported by arms or straps if necessary. Her feet should be flat on the floor, or, if this is not possible, resting on a box. Most importantly, the table should be at the level of her waist, so that she can comfortably rest her elbows on the table. A child who can hardly see over the edge of the table is going to have a tough time learning to feed herself.

Feeding herself

Teaching a child to feed herself is done most easily if the teacher stands behind the child: what is lost in face-to-face contact is made up for in the natural flow of the teacher's movements guiding the child's hand.

In general it seems best to start teaching the child to feed herself with foods that she is very, very fond of. If she loves pudding but only tolerates meat and vegetables, we feed her her first course as usual and start the teaching with the pudding. If the food she is really mad about is ice-cream then we have ice-cream for pudding for a few days. When she begins to get the hang of feeding herself she can go on to foods that she likes but which are not her first favourite.

1. Finger feeding

To teach this we take a suitable food that the child likes and cut it up into pieces or lengths: apple, banana, biscuits, bread and butter or toast and spreads, celery, carrot, fried bread, sweets such as barley sugar, rusks, are all possible. Standing behind the child, we close her fingers round a piece and move her hand up to her mouth. We encourage her to smell the food, touch it with her lips and tongue, to put it into her mouth and taste it. Gradually, as she begins to hold and move the food to her mouth herself we relax our pressure.

2. Using a spoon

Sometimes a child is slow in learning to feed herself because it doesn't occur to her family to let her try to feed herself: in other cases she actively resists the process. With some children it may be helpful to put a tiny blob of a favourite food – jam, syrup, melted chocolate, a smear of Marmite – onto the tip of the spoon, give the child a taste of it, and then let her try by herself taking the spoon to her mouth. Later she may be willing to take the spoon with tiny portions of dinner on it to her mouth.

Other children, however, will not take the spoon to their mouths at all. Karen was one of these; she was pleased to get her food as long as her mother fed it to her, but as soon as she was given a spoon she would open her hand and drop it, and if her mother returned it to her she got cross and threw it away. When Karen was four, and obviously perfectly capable of

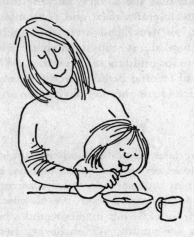

feeding herself, her mother decided it was time for her to begin doing so. For the first attempt her mother made her favourite dinner – sausage, mashed potatoes and carrots. She cut the sausage and carrots up into small pieces and poured over some of Karen's favourite gravy. She popped Karen into her high chair and put on a good-sized plastic bib. She put the plate in front of Karen, loaded the spoon with a small quantity of sausage and potato, and, standing behind the high chair, put Karen's hand round the handle of the spoon: with her own hand round Karen's she guided the spoon to Karen's mouth. Karen resisted holding the spoon, but as her mother's hand held hers firmly round the handle she could not drop it, and she was really pleased to get such a nice mouthful of food. Her mother guided the spoon back to the plate, gave Karen a little hug and said to her, 'What a clever girl! You did it yourself!' Then she scooped up another small spoonful of food and, when Karen had finished her mouthful, they were ready to start again.

As Karen was so resistant her mother did not at first insist on her feeding herself the whole meal. Instead she stopped after the first three mouthfuls, and fed Karen the rest of the meal as she had always done. They went on like this for three or four meals, and then Karen's mother increased the number of spoonfuls Karen 'fed herself' to four, later to six, eight, eleven, and so on, until eventually Karen was expected to help with the whole course. This was the normal way of things, but her mother would not expect Karen to do so much if she were unwell or upset or if the meal were something she was not so keen on. Never again, however, did Karen get away with having the whole meal fed to her.

As Karen began to be more skilful at using her spoon her mother began to fade out the help she was giving her. At first she slightly released her hold just as the spoon reached Karen's lips, so that Karen did more of the action of putting the bowl of the spoon into her mouth; she did not let go of Karen's hand entirely, and it was just as well she did not because when Karen had got the mouthful of food she forthwith lost interest in holding the spoon and would have dropped it if her mother had not made sure that she replaced it decorously on the plate. Later on her mother was able to release Karen's hand earlier and earlier in the process of taking the spoon from the plate to her mouth, and eventually gradually to release her hold of Karen's hand, until she was not actually touching Karen's hand at all. The first time she let go altogether of Karen's hand she was so delighted that she stood back to enjoy the sight of her daughter feeding herself – whereupon Karen dropped the spoon. Karen's mother retrieved the spoon from the floor, gave it a wash, and decided that she should not be quite so precipitate next time; when she next let go of Karen's hand she kept her hand hovering just above Karen's, shadowing her movements, so that if Karen showed any sign of making a mistake her mother was right there to help.

Karen made good progress with learning to take the spoonful of food to her mouth – probably because she liked the food; the reinforcement was there for her at the end of the spoon-lifting process. It was more difficult to teach her to put the spoon back on her plate – probably because there was not much reinforcement in that. Her mother decided that Karen would be more likely to learn to put down her spoon properly if she were reinforced for doing so. As her mouth was always full with her last spoonful of food her mother could not use a food reinforcer; instead, when the spoon reached the plate her mother would praise her and gently stroke her cheek, which Karen loved. With this and the gradual fading of her mother's prompts she learnt to return her spoon to the plate.

Another difficult task was loading the spoon. Her mother did not start teaching this until Karen was well on the way to being able to take the spoon to her mouth. Then her mother collected the food to one side of the plate before giving the spoon to Karen, putting her hand round Karen's and helping her to scoop up a spoonful of food. Later, when Karen was beginning to be able to do the scooping her mother prompted her to scrape the food together.

3. *Using a fork*

When Karen was able to use a spoon with little help her mother put a fork into her left hand and prompted her to use it to push the food into the spoon. Her mother thought that, occupying her left hand, the fork would help to discourage Karen from using her fingers. Occasionally in the past Karen would use her fingers to push food on to the spoon, so here the fork was of practical help as well as socially more acceptable.

Once again Karen's mother gradually faded out her prompts, taking care not to go too quickly, until Karen could manage the fork by herself.

4. *Using a knife*

When her mother wanted to teach Karen to cut with a knife she began teaching her as part of a game, which they played in playtime, quite apart from meal times. Together they cut Plasticine, clay and dough, with her mother prompting Karen to hold and move the knife with her right hand and to hold whatever she was cutting with her left hand. Later they started cutting bread with the crusts off at tea-time: at the same time, and using the same methods of prompting and fading, her mother taught Karen to spread soft butter and jam on the bread.

A good deal later, when Karen had for some months been able to use a spoon and fork quite by herself, her mother began to teach her to cut foods such as bananas, fish fingers, soft buns, cooked carrots, pears, tinned peaches and so on with a knife while holding the food steady with a fork. She then encouraged Karen to put the food into her mouth with the fork. (This was quite a big change for Karen as up to now she had taken the food to her mouth in a spoon held in her right hand, whereas the fork now was in her left hand.) Her mother made a point of showing Karen how to cut the food with a forward and backward movement of the knife; so when she came to use her knife at dinner she could cut her meat instead of trying to wrench it apart sideways.

5. *Drinking from a cup*

When we want to teach a child to drink by herself the kind of cup we use depends on what she finds easiest. Some children do best with a beaker without handles, for others a two-handled cup is good (see Appendix 4, 'Aids and Equipment'). For very young children the Trainer Beakers are excellent and save spilling. Whichever kind of cup you choose, fill it with a drink the child likes and about half full – more and it is likely to slop about, less and the child has to tip it so far to get anything as to make the task extra difficult. We put the child's hands on to the cup: even if she is using a one-handled cup the hand on the other side will help to steady it. We help her to pick the cup up to her lips, tip it so that she gets a little of the drink, and then put the cup down again. Gradually, as she begins to be able to do some of the task herself we fade the prompts.

Once again, as with the spoon, the most difficult part to teach is putting the cup back on the table, and it may help if we reinforce this part of the task separately. We shadow the child's hands carefully at this stage so that she can't drop the cup or spill the drink.

Managing and taking foods

1. *Chewing*

It is difficult to teach this, especially with an older child, and we may have to be persistent. Try offering, or getting her to take to her mouth, long pieces of food so that she can bite them, hopefully bite them off, with her front teeth. Try any of the foods listed under 'Finger feeding' (see page 153). To control her lips and jaw we stand behind her, put a middle finger below and forefinger above her lips, and the rest of our fingers under her chin: then we rub the thumb, and fingers of the other hand, gently round the outside of her cheeks to encourage chewing with her back teeth. We can also gently move her jaw up and down – not too hard or she may bite her tongue or cheeks.

You can get more help from Jennifer Warner's *Helping the Handicapped Child with Early Feeding*, from which the suggestions above were taken (see Appendix 3).

2. *Going from smooth to thicker to lumpy foods*

This problem often goes with the last. Children who can't chew will only take very smooth liquidized food – or else it is that children who will only take smooth foods never learn to chew. Whichever way round, the time comes when the child should get on to thicker foods as a first step towards ordinary foods. Carol (page 86) at the age of ten would take only liquid food and only out of a bottle. She was a big girl, and quite active, and it looked absolutely ridiculous for her to be sitting up at table drinking from a bottle, and so her teacher decided to try to teach her to take more normal food. First, Carol had to be persuaded to drink out of a cup. Next her favourite milk drink was made very slightly thicker by adding a little cornflour to it. When she would take that well it was made a little thicker still. At the same time she began to have other foods, meat, fish and vegetables, at first liquidized to a consistency of thin cream but later becoming rather thicker by leaving out some of the liquid.

When her teacher wanted Carol to begin to take lumpy foods she started off by introducing very tiny lumps – half grains of cooked rice – into the milk drinks. She also began to teach Carol to eat from a spoon, giving her the first two or three mouthfuls from a spoon before allowing her to have the rest from a cup. This programme is still going on. The most difficult part is with the lumps: as soon as Carol finds a lump larger than a cooked grain of rice she spits it out. So it looks as if it is going to be a long job to get her to eat ordinary food like anyone else.

Since it is so difficult to persuade older children to accept foods of different textures, especially if they have always been used to a smooth liquid diet, it is important to introduce thicker, lumpy foods to children while they are young – if possible under a year. This difficulty with food textures seems to occur particularly with children with visual handicaps, though we don't know why.

3. *Taking new or disliked foods*

If a child is suspicious of trying new foods we offer her a very small amount of it at first, following it up with a spoonful of something she does like. Much the same approach can be tried if a child particularly dislikes a food which it is important that she should eat – one or two food fads are permissible, dozens are not. Simon (page 75) would eat only potato, toast, fish fingers, mince, milk, baked beans, mousse and ice-cream. He would not eat eggs, meat (apart from mince), fruit, vegetables or salads, and suffered badly from constipation. His teacher decided to try to teach him to take a variety of foods. At first he had to touch a piece of, say, carrot with his tongue: later he had to touch it with his lips, then take it into his mouth, then chew, and later still swallow it, in order to gain his reinforcement – a Smartie. It sounds weird, giving a child sweets in the middle of his dinner, rewarding him with choco-late for swallowing a piece of cauliflower, and many people said it would never work: but it did. You couldn't really say that Simon now eats a normal diet but he eats a great many things – eggs, bacon, meat, and some vegetables – that he never did before.

In the same way if a child loves her pudding and dislikes her first course it may be worth rewarding her with a spoonful of the pudding for taking a spoonful of the first course. Later she may have to take two spoonfuls of the first course, then three, and so on, in order to get her spoonful of pudding. And if the idea of toad-in-the-hole alternating with chocolate mousse makes you shudder, but it works, then you should, as my son said on a quite different occasion, try not to think about it.

Table manners

Besides teaching a child how to feed herself we may also want to teach her good table manners. This may make all the difference between people being pleased to have her at meals with them and not being willing to sit down at table with her. For Owen it meant the difference between being taken on family excursions and being left behind. 'Before, he was so awful we didn't dare take him to a restaurant, but now – well, we had lunch in a restaurant on Friday and he was fine, and we all enjoyed it.'

We teach table manners by prompting the good behaviour, where necessary; reinforcing it by praise and by allowing the child to continue eating; and sometimes discouraging the bad behaviour by, for instance, interrupting her eating. It is impor-tant to be very consistent in our teaching so that the child does not learn that she can occasionally get away with bad manners.

Later we have to fade out the supervision while still making sure she does not slip back into bad habits.

1. *Using fingers*

Some foods, like biscuits and sandwiches, can and should be eaten with fingers: others, like stew, mashed potato and jelly, should not. Sometimes children prefer to use their fingers, especially when they are not very skilful with a spoon and can get the food more easily with their fingers. To avoid this we try to keep the hand not holding the spoon busy, prompting it to hold a fork, or the side of the plate, or perhaps just to stay on the child's lap. If the child does use her fingers we say 'No' and remove her plate for ten seconds. Then we wipe her fingers if they are messy, give her back her spoon, re-occupy her other hand, and try again.

2. *Troughing or pigging*

These picturesque terms refer to eating straight from the plate with the mouth, without benefit of fingers or cutlery. Again, we say 'No' and remove the plate. Before we give it back again we make sure the child is sitting up straight, lifting her chin with our hand if necessary. Her seating position is important here; a child whose chin is only just over the table top is more likely to lapse into troughing than one whose position puts her at the proper height above the table.

3. *Bolting food*

Sometimes a child will gobble down her food, perhaps without chewing it. If telling her to eat more slowly does not have any effect we may try taking her plate away between mouthfuls. Another method, used with Trevor (page 94), was to take away the plate for ten seconds every time he tried to put in another mouthful before he had swallowed the last. Another method to try is gently to hold down the child's arm when she tries to gobble – this, like taking away the plate, means that she gets her food more slowly than if she were eating properly: so she learns that she actually gets more food in a shorter time if she eats properly.

4. *Snatching food from somebody else's plate*

We try not to let the child benefit from her snatching – that is, we try to get the food she snatched away from her before she can eat it. Then we take away her plate, if there is anything on it, for ten seconds.

5. *Throwing food and tipping over plates*

Sometimes a child seems to do this when she has had enough to eat but is urged to take some more. In this case perhaps we should be more ready to accept her signals. If she pushes her plate away we ask her if she wants some more, and if she pushes it away again remove her plate.

In other circumstances, if she throws food or tips over her plate out of temper, or, perhaps, to make us cross, we take her food away and don't give her any more. Any food we remove should be firmly thrown away. It seems wasteful at the time, but if we can teach the child to eat properly we will probably waste less in the end.

Of course if the child spills her food or drink by accident we clear it up without making a fuss.

6. *Slowness over eating*

Sometimes a child, far from bolting her food, is so slow over eating that the meals almost merge into each other. How we deal with this will depend partly on why she is so slow, and partly on how she feels about her food. Terry, who was 14, was fond of his food but seemed to have got into the habit of lingering over it, to put it mildly. He was told that he would be allowed the following times to eat his meals:

Breakfast:

cereal:	10 minutes
hot dish:	15 ,,
bread and butter:	10 ,,

Mid-day meal:

meat and vegetable:	20 minutes
sweet:	10 ,,

When a course was given to him a kitchen timer was set to go off at the end of the allotted period, and he was told that anything he had not finished when the timer rang would be thrown away. No particular notice was taken of Terry during this time, he was not urged to hurry or warned about how much time had gone by. When the timer rang, his plate was removed and the food thrown away, and, in spite of his protests, Terry was never given any extra time. When he finished within the time he was praised. Terry soon learnt to finish within the time allowed. After this the timer, although still set, was moved away where he could not see it; he still managed to finish within the time so the programme was discontinued. Three months later he was still eating at a normal speed.

Terry seemed to enjoy the challenge of 'Beat the Clock' but other children may need some other reinforcement for their success. Maisie, for example, was allowed a comic to look at whenever she completed her meal on time. As with all the programmes there is no hard and fast rule: what we do depends on the individual child we are working with, how we run the programme depends on how the child responds to it.

The main points

1. Teaching feeding is often enjoyable because food is reinforcing to most children.

2. It is important that the child should be seated in a correct position.

3. Self-feeding:
   (a) We stand behind the child to teach her;
   (b) We begin by using foods she likes;
   (c) We use prompting, fading and backward chaining;
   (d) We don't fade prompts too quickly;
   (e) In spoon-feeding, we teach and reinforce putting the spoon back on the plate separately;
   (f) We use games to teach cutting with a knife, encouraging a sawing movement;
   (g) In teaching drinking we teach and reinforce separately putting the cup down.

4. Managing and taking foods:
   (a) We introduce new textures of food very gradually;
   (b) We offer new foods, or those the child dislikes, in very small quantities, alternating them with something the child does like.

5. Table manners:
   (a) If a child enjoys her food, her plate may be taken away for a short time (10 seconds) if she:
   uses her fingers;
   troughs (make her sit upright);
   snatches (don't let her eat what she has snatched).
   (b) Bolting food: we take the plate away between mouthfuls, or hold her arm down when she tries to gobble.
   (c) Throwing and tipping plates: we take away the child's food and don't give any more.
   (d) Slowness: we give the child a certain time to finish her food, don't nag her to hurry or give her extra time.

Some practice problems

*1. Suppose you were a Chinese parent. How would you set about teaching a child to use chopsticks? (Aren't you glad you don't have to!)

*2. Make a list of foods that we sometimes eat with our fingers, sometimes with cutlery. How would you teach a child when she should use one and when the other?

*3. How would you teach a child to set a table?

*4. Lucy can feed herself very well but as soon as she has finished eating as much as she wants she tips the plate over – not, apparently, to be tiresome but to show that she has had enough. How would you deal with this?

12. Play

Play is one of the most important parts of a child's life. Besides helping her to learn useful things like positioning, turning and balancing things and how the action of one thing affects another, and besides stretching her imagination and learning give and take with other children, play occupies the child. When she plays she is busy and happy and does not need constant attention from other people; her parents can have a few blessed moments to themselves. Some children with learning disabilities do not know how to play; so we try to teach them.

There are three main kinds of play:

1. Play with toys.
2. Social play (playing with other children).
3. Imaginative play.

1. Play with toys

Most children spend much of their time playing with toys, and indeed with anything else they can get hold of – sugar-bowls, saucepans, the contents of Mum's handbag, and so on. Some children with learning disabilities, however, do not play with toys, and instead may spend their free time doing things they shouldn't. Others may have a special affection for one particular toy which they refuse to be parted from, and it is often hard to persuade these children to play with anything else, especially if they become upset when the 'special' toy is removed. Other children again are interested in toys but treat them so badly, throwing or breaking them, that they have to be taken away from them. These problems will be discussed in a moment.

PLAY 167

Why is toy-play important?

For many children play is the thing they do most of the time.
When they play with toys they take in all kinds of information
about their surroundings, and about themselves. For example,
when building a tower out of bricks the child learns how to
pick up a brick, how to let go of it, how to make her hand
move the brick a little to the right or left according to what her
eyes tell her so that the tower will not fall over; she learns how
balancing the bricks gets harder the higher the tower, what
happens when the top brick is not on quite straight, what
happens when you pull out a brick at the bottom of the tower,
and so on. This kind of learning is important for her development, and play with toys (or objects) teaches her skills which
are useful to her later on. So it is especially important for
children with learning disabilities to learn to play, since
they of all people need to learn as many useful skills as possible.

Another powerful reason for teaching play is that children
with learning disabilities should be taught, whenever possible,
to do anything that other children do. Another reason for most
parents is the need to be able to leave their learning-disabled
child to occupy herself for short periods of time: a child who
cannot occupy herself even for a minute is unbelievably wearing to be with.

Selecting toys

Before embarking on ways of teaching a child to play with toys
we should think about what toys to give her. Two things
should be taken into account – the things she likes, and the
level of development she has reached.

What she likes

The more fascinating a toy is to a child the more she is going
to play with it (with or without help), so we want to choose

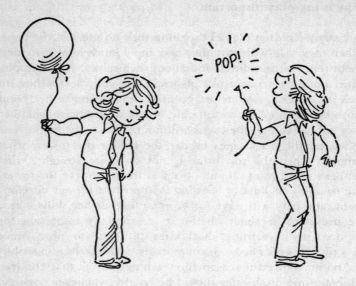

toys that she will specially like. If she does not at present play with toys at all we can see what sort of everyday things she likes, and how these could be included in a toy for her. If she loves noise, then (provided of course that we can stand the row) we should choose noisy toys – squeezy animals with a very loud squeak, pegs to be hammered into holes, posting boxes where the shape makes a noise when it falls through the hole, and so on. There are a great many toys available now which give the child feedback – provide a reaction to her action: she presses a button and a face pops up, pushes a switch and music plays, bangs a knob and a figure shoots out of its hole. We can select a toy which accords with the child's particular interests so that it is likely to be reinforcing to her and, of itself, will hold her attention. In this way we can choose the toys that are likely to be the best ones for her. At first it may be best to borrow toys from a toy library if you have one in your area. They are now called Toy and Leisure Libraries, and there are over 1,000 distributed over the country. Toys can be borrowed from them, some charging a small annual subscription and some a small borrowing fee but many lending out the toys free of charge. Toy library staff are extremely helpful about choosing the right toy for a child, and can often suggest ways to encourage her to play with and enjoy it, and they are understanding about breakages. So by borrowing toys from the library we can see which toys appeal to the child before going to the expense of buying them. The National Association of Toy and Leisure Libraries will always be pleased to put you in touch with your local library (see Appendix 2).

Age level

It can be difficult to choose toys that are neither too easy nor too difficult for a child, especially if she is good at some things but poor at others. Children who like toys usually push aside those that are too easy or too difficult. However, when a child is not very interested in toys at all it is difficult to get much guidance from her behaviour with toys as to which are roughly at her level. In this case it is worth asking the child's teacher, or the local psychologist if there is one, or the toy library staff, for advice. If all else fails we just have to try out some toys at random. We start with easy toys, as we can always move on to harder ones, whereas starting with toys that are too hard can be discouraging. The parents of most children (I, for one) tend to buy toys that are too difficult so that the children only begin to play with the toys months later, by which time they are no longer excitingly new. Since it is obviously easy to over-estimate a child's level, it seems best to start with toys which might be below rather than above that level.

The following is a very rough guide to toys for each age level. (See Appendix 3 for more comprehensive guides to toys for different age groups.) With a learning-disabled child we cannot always go by how old she is, but rather by the age her kind of behaviour suggests. For example an 8-year-old child might be doing things more like a 3-year-old. In this case some of the toys for her are listed under the 3-year age group.

Age	Toys
0–6 months	Rattles, bells, mobiles, mirrors, own hands, odd items to look at, hold, mouth and so on.
6–12 months	Toys that wobble (e.g. those on suction pads), noisy toys (that squeak), bells and rattles, pull-along toys, big building bricks, odd items (cups, spoons, etc.).
12–18 months	Posting boxes (simple ones, single or 2-hole), form-boards (few pieces only), stacking toys (can't do it by size though), building bricks, peg-boards, crayons (scribble and strokes, not pictures), balls, hammer and peg toys, sand and water play, picture books (looking at pictures).
18 months–2 years	3–4-hole posting boxes, form-boards and stacking toys, hammer and peg toys, crayons (beginning to imitate strokes), picture books (beginning to understand names of objects in pictures, and names a few), building bricks, cars and dolls, soft toys.
2–3 years	Multi-hole posting boxes, form-boards and stacking toys, paper cutting and sticking, threading, colour matching, simple constructional toys, crayons and paints, picture books.
3–4 years	Simple jig-saws (up to 6 pieces), complex form-boards, crayons and pencils (beginning to copy simple things), simple picture matching, constructional toys, doll's houses, cutting and sticking.

Teaching children to play with toys

Learning how to use toys

Denis was 5 years old and very, very active. He spent his time at home rushing up and down the stairs, jumping on the beds, galloping round the garden, turning chairs over, and so on. He showed no interest in toys, except occasionally to put them in his mouth and blow them out on to a hard surface (making a good bang), and he could not be left alone to play because he would throw the toys and upset the furniture.

Careful observation of Denis suggested that most of his troublesome behaviour was due to over-activity and to his liking for noise – part of the fun of overturning furniture seemed to be the noise it made. So it was decided that Denis should be taught to play properly with some very simple toys, with the aim that eventually he would play with them for a short time by himself. The toys chosen were simple stacking toys, a simple posting box and a hammer toy in which balls were banged through holes with a hammer.

His teacher had five-minute sessions with Denis, as often as she could manage it. She sat him at a table during these sessions, and taught one toy at a time. With the stacking toy she prompted him to stack one ring on another, with her hands moving Denis's hands to pick up the ring and put it on another. Then she reinforced him, giving him a kiss and a jelly-tot (which he loved). The prompts were gradually faded until Denis could do the stacking toy with only slight prompts and eventually without any at all. At this stage he would stack one ring on another, get reinforcement, then stack another ring and get reinforcement, and so on. He could not get the sizes of the graduated rings right, but if the rings were laid out in the right order he could put them on correctly. In the same way Denis learnt to hammer the balls through the holes, and to post the shapes through the posting box. He could not match lots of different shapes to holes, so very simple one-shape and then two-shape posting boxes were used.

It took several months to teach Denis this much. Now his teacher, and his mother who is doing the same thing at home, give him reinforcement every second time he puts on a ring, hammers a ball through or posts a shape; soon they will move on to reinforcing him every third time, and so on. Eventually when he can do the tasks completely – stack all the rings or bang all the balls through – for one reinforcement it should be possible to begin to get him to play alone (like Olga, see page 173). Since he is so fond of noise it seems likely that out of the three toys he has learnt to use the one he will most successfully

play alone with is the hammer toy, just because this is likely to
be the one he will enjoy most.

Denis is fairly typical of the child who shows no interest in
ordinary toys, although his energy and activity probably made
Denis more of a menace than most. The methods his teacher
used are suitable for most children: we choose a small number
of toys of the right level, and then use *prompting* and *fading*
(pages 61–6), *backward chaining* (see page 67) and *reinforcement* (see pages 25–39) to teach the child to play with each toy.
Once he can play with these toys it should be a little easier to
teach him to go on to play with other toys; though, as he may
not spontaneously generalize his play (see pages 73–5), he may
need more teaching whenever he meets new toys.

Playing with new toys

Timmy was like Denis in that he showed no interest in ordinary
toys (see page 33). However, he did have a special toy from
which he would not be parted, a small plastic cup which he
hung over his thumb and twiddled. It became known as
'Timmy's twiddler' and it would keep him 'occupied' for
hours. The trouble was that while he twiddled he could not
learn anything new; he just was not interested in other things
while he had his twiddler. If, on the other hand, the cup was
taken away from him he would scream and pull at his hair and
face until the cup was returned to him. (Timmy punished
people for removing his cup by screaming and pulling his hair,
which they hated: while anybody who returned his cup was
negatively reinforced by his stopping the screaming and hair-
pulling.) One way and another Timmy had taught people not
to take away his cup.

If Timmy were to learn anything it would be necessary to
remove his twiddler, despite his protests. So his teacher decided to start removing the twiddler for very short periods and
to begin teaching him to play with toys. The teaching methods
were identical with those used with Denis, except that during
the teaching part while Timmy had no twiddler he tended to

enliven the session with screams of protest (his hands were being prompted through the required actions and so he had no chance to pull at his hair or face). The reinforcer for Timmy was the twiddler; each time he had done what was wanted of him his teacher gave him back his twiddler for about ten or twenty seconds. Timmy gradually learnt the routine, and, after he had done what was wanted, would reach out his hand for his twiddler. Since he was never now given back his twiddler when he screamed or pulled his hair, but was only given it when he was not doing these things he also learnt to scream and pull his hair less. He has never learnt not to scream or pull his hair at all, but perhaps this was because he was about 12 years old when the teaching started so that these were long-standing habits. Similarly, although it was possible to teach him to play to some extent with a few toys, he never learnt to play with them alone.

Timmy is a good example of a child who is so attached to one toy that he will not willingly play with any other. Many of these children make much more progress than Timmy did; it depends a great deal on how able the child is and how devoted to the special toy. Other ways of dealing with things the child is very strongly attached to are discussed in chapter 13, 'Getting Over Phobias and Obsessions'.

Playing alone

Olga was 11 and could play with simple toys but would never play by herself. As soon as her mother left the room Olga would get up and follow her and pester her with questions, leaving the toys behind. Her mother's observations showed that, left to herself, Olga would play for up to five minutes with water (pouring, tipping, emptying and filling containers), for less than a minute with a simple form-board, and for less than two minutes with stacking rings. If her mother or father sat next to her Olga would play for a good deal longer.

It was decided that Olga should have two kinds of teaching sessions; one to teach her to play with new toys, using the same methods as those used for Denis, and the other to teach her to play on her own with toys she was used to. In this second programme Olga was given one of her own toys to play with and her mother then moved quietly away to the other side of the room. After a short time (about half a minute) she went over to Olga and, if she was still playing, reinforced her with praise and a drink. If Olga had stopped playing she was not reinforced but was told to go on with her playing. These sessions only lasted about ten minutes, and the time between reinforcements was gradually lengthened (over the weeks) from every half a minute to every few minutes. A few months later Olga's mother found she could withdraw for quite a few minutes to another room and Olga would continue playing on her own. She did of course still need to help Olga to learn to play with new toys, but it was nice for Olga (and for her mother) that she could now play on her own with toys that she knew well.

This kind of programme, with perhaps small changes to suit different children, should be useful for most of those who are already able to play with some simple toys and who need to learn to play without supervision. Children are usually more willing to play alone with simple toys which they know well than with more advanced toys, so it is a good idea to teach a child to occupy herself using toys that are well within her range. We can then teach her to play with more advanced toys in separate sessions, as Olga's mother did. When these have been mastered then of course they can be used in the 'playing alone' times too.

Playing properly

Duncan was $2\frac{1}{2}$ years old and, on the whole, very well behaved. However, when he had toys within reach he would pick them up in turn and throw them round the room. His parents would scold him and pick the toys up for him. In the baseline observations ten toys were given to him ten times each, and the average length of time he held the toys before throwing them was found to be six and a half seconds. Each time Duncan threw a toy he looked round to see what his parents' reactions were; it seemed that he threw his toys partly to get their attention. So it was decided that his parents would treat his throwing by *extinction* (see page 88) – that is, they would no longer scold him, or pick up the toys, or pay any attention at all to his throwing. In addition, since Duncan seemed not to know what he *should* be doing with the toys, his parents taught him, in quite short sessions of about five minutes at a time, how to play properly with the toys. The reinforcers that they used were praise and clapping; these, as we might have expected (because Duncan had already shown that he was eager for his parents' attention), were very good reinforcers for him. The result was that within about eight weeks Duncan was holding his toys and playing with them for an average of about one minute instead of six and a half seconds, and beaming all over his face whenever he was praised or clapped. His playing continued to improve over the next months and Duncan was transformed from a little terror in the playroom to a boy whom it was a pleasure to have around.

Duncan did not play with toys properly because he had unintentionally been reinforced, by all the attention his parents gave him, when he threw them. Children like Duncan often improve rapidly once the wrong kind of play is no longer reinforced. It is a good idea also to do as Duncan's parents did, and teach and reinforce the proper ways of playing with toys, since it may be quite difficult for the children to learn this of their own accord. Then the reinforcement given for the proper play takes the place of the reinforcement that used to be given for the wrong kind of play; which means that the child gets at least as much of the good things in life as before.

2. Social play: playing with other children

Most very young children take relatively little notice of each other when playing, but by about the age of 2 they begin to play alongside other children. Gradually between about 2 and 3 years old, they begin to respond more and more to each other and to play together. Children probably learn a lot about getting along with other people through play – how to take turns, how to be a leader at one time and a follower at another, how to be friendly and how to cope with unfriendliness.

Some learning-disabled children do not play cooperatively with other children and we may want to teach them to do so. It may be easier to teach this in school, where there are plenty of other children around, than at home, where there may be only one or two brothers or sisters. Nevertheless, if we want to we can make a start on teaching cooperative play at home, using a brother or sister (as in the example of Robin on page 177) or perhaps a neighbour's friendly child. Here again suitable toys can help. Some toys such as see-saws, and most ball games, need more than one player to play them, as do many of the table-top games such as snap or snakes and ladders. So these are good ones to choose for teaching a child to play with others, especially if we think the child would enjoy them. Which ones we choose will of course depend partly on the child's ability – see-saws and simple ball games come at the lower end of the scale. Many other toys can with a little ingenuity be turned into social games; for instance doing a jigsaw can be a social affair if each child has half the pieces and they have to take turns to put pieces in. This can be an especially useful thing to do if, for instance, the child does not like the kinds of things which need two people to do them, like see-saws, but does enjoy jigsaws.

Very simple social play

Sometimes a child will not play with other children because she is not interested in contacts with people at all, neither with adults nor with other children. If we want to teach her to play, perhaps as a step towards her making and enjoying contacts with others, then the play will have to be very simple – rolling a ball or playing (with help) a simple table game like snap with another child, or sitting on a see-saw with another child at the other end, each helping to make the see-saw work. Teaching this kind of play will probably need, first, a cooperative second child as helper; and second, prompting and reinforcement of 'playfulness' in the child being taught. Deliberate reinforcement of the child's play may need to be continued for quite some time, as if it is stopped she might stop being willing to play. But if reinforcement is given over and over again alongside the social happenings going on at the same time – contacts with the other children, praise and encouragement from them perhaps – then eventually these social happenings themselves may become reinforcing. If they do, the child has taken a big step forward.

Responding to children as well as adults

Some children only find pleasure in contacts with adults, and not in contacts with other children such as brothers and sisters. Where a child responds to adult praise, hugs, cuddles and so on it is as a rule not so hard to teach her to play with other children, usually by reinforcing the play with adult attention.

Four-year-old Robin managed to get his parents' attention in various devious ways, such as turning up the volume on the radio or television, swinging on the curtains, turning on taps in the kitchen and, when all else failed, kicking or pinching his 6-year-old sister. Robin's sister was a kind and patient girl who never retaliated, but just endured her brother's assaults. Whenever Robin attacked her their parents would give Robin 'a good talking to' but Robin seemed oblivious to the niceties of the concept of 'fair play' and, as time went on, he bothered his sister more rather than less. Fortunately Robin adored doing simple jigsaws which his mother normally helped him with. So now she decided that both she and Robin's sister would help Robin with his jigsaws, each of them praising and petting him for a good performance. Gradually Robin's mother began to withdraw for a short time (just a few seconds at first), returning every now and again to reinforce Robin before withdrawing again. Robin's sister also gave reinforcement, praising and petting him as she had seen her mother do, and eventually, after weeks of sessions, Robin's mother did not need to return at all during the ten-minute sessions. Then other games were introduced, in which Robin's sister could take more part, such as constructional toys. Although Robin's sister never really enjoyed the games (they were rather young for her) she did begin to like the sessions because Robin's obvious enjoyment of them was reinforcing to her, and moreover she no longer got bitten and kicked. Robin, for his part, had learnt to play cooperatively with at least one person.

3. Imaginative play

Much of an older child's play involves representation: things stand for other things, as when doll's house furniture stands for real furniture, or children stand for other people when they dress up as nurses or cowboys. Imaginative play is an important part of a child's development, although its place in her development is not altogether clear. Some experts feel that imaginative play comes before and helps the development of language: others, that language comes before imaginative play, which just reflects a high level of language development. Either way, most children do not show a lot of imaginative play until they have a good deal of understanding of language, and it is not easy to teach imaginative play to children who are showing no signs of understanding or using language.

In the few cases where people have tried to teach children imaginative play they have usually found that although they could teach the child one particular play, such as pouring imaginary tea from a teapot and pretending to drink it, the child did not go on to play new imaginary games on her own. In other words the child did not generalize (see page 73). So it is perhaps not worth trying to teach imaginative play to a child who shows no signs that she is ready for it. If, on the other hand, a child is teetering on the brink of imaginative play – cuddling dollies, or putting a teddy to bed occasionally – we should certainly reinforce such play and provide suitable things for the child to play with. Certain kinds of equipment – cars and garages, dolls, doll's prams and houses, tea-sets, play houses, and all kinds of clothes for dressing up – can act as cues for imaginative play. If we provide these kinds of materials the child will be more likely to play imaginatively, especially if we help her by playing the games with her.

The main points

1. Playing with toys is an important way for the child to learn new things.

2. We should choose toys which suit the level of development the child has reached, and those that are likely to have a particular appeal for the child.

3. A child who likes a toy is more likely to learn to play with it.

4. To teach a child to play with toys we use reinforcement (chapter 3) and prompting, fading and backward chaining (chapter 5).

5. The best reinforcement for play comes from the toy itself; if reinforcement has to be given by the teacher it must continue to be given until the child finds the toy reinforcing in itself.

6. A 'special' toy which the child is very attached to can be used as a reinforcer.

7. Once a child can play with some simple toys, she can be taught to play on her own, usually by 'fading out' the adult helper.

8. If we get rid of a bad behaviour with toys we may still have to teach the child to play properly with the toys.

9. Children can be encouraged to play with other children if the right sort of toys are available.

10. Children who do not play with other children may be either:

 (a) quite uninterested in the company and reactions of people; these children can be taught only simple social play, using deliberately provided reinforcement; or

 (b) reinforced only by adult company and reactions; if these are first paired with responses from other children, and then faded out, these children may come to enjoy being with other children.

11. Imaginative play cannot easily be taught to children with little or no language.

12. We can encourage imaginative play by providing the right kind of materials and reinforcing the right kind of play.

Some practice problems

 1. What toys do your children find reinforcing?

*2. What kinds of toys do you think blind children might find reinforcing, or deaf/blind children?

*3. How could you teach a child not to keep asking, 'Mum, I'm fed up – what can I do?'?

*4. What would you do if you wanted to teach a child to play with other children when the child in question actually *avoids* other children and becomes upset if other children approach, but she does find adult attention reinforcing?

13. Getting Over Phobias and Obsessions

Phobias

Sometimes children develop fears that are quite out of proportion to the dangerousness of the things they are afraid of. Simon was so frightened of having a bath that for six years he refused to have one at all (see page 133). Andy (see page 97) was terrified of dogs and could not stay in the room with the smallest chihuahua. Dino went into a panic if anyone attempted to touch his legs (see pages 184–6). Other children have been afraid of going in cars, sitting on lavatories, getting dirt on their clothes, having their hair washed, going into large shops and many other things which in themselves are not dangerous.

These fears are quite common too in other children, and in adults. Just why they develop is not always clear. Sometimes there may be an obvious reason; sometimes we can guess at one. Claire's parents (see page 186) wondered whether she had ever been hurt by uncomfortable shoes, but they could not pin it down to anything definite. Sometimes, as in the case of Matthew, there seems to be no imaginable reason for the fears (page 190). But not knowing why the problem arose does not mean that it cannot be dealt with.

The methods used to help children with learning disabilities to get over their fears are much the same as those used for other people; the two main ones are called *graded practice* and *flooding*.

Graded practice

The object of this method is gradually to accustom the child to what she fears, starting at the point where she is hardly afraid at all and gradually working up to the point that she needs to reach – where her ordinary life can go on without being disrupted by her fears. We begin by making a list of the things the child finds frightening, starting at the lowest level, with aspects of the thing that she finds not frightening at all. For example, although Andy was frightened of any real dog he was not at all frightened of stuffed toy dogs. Next on the list come aspects of the thing that the child finds very, very slightly worrying: in Andy's case large lifelike models of dogs. So we move very gradually up the scale until we come to the aspect of the thing that the child is likely to have to cope with in ordinary life. In Andy's case this was friendly dogs of any size quite close to him; this was what he was likely to meet in the streets and shops and people's homes. This list of aspects of the feared thing, graded very carefully in very small steps from the least frightening to the most-frightening-necessary is called a *hierarchy*.

So for Andy his hierarchy of 'dog-frighteningness' went as follows:

1. Stuffed toy dog
2. Model of a small dog
3. Model of a large dog
4. Film of a small dog in the background
5. Film of a small dog in the foreground
6. Film of a small dog in close-up
7. Film of a large dog in the background
8. Film of a large dog in the foreground
9. Film of a large dog in close-up
10. Small dog behind a wire fence, 3 metres away
11. Large dog behind a wire fence, 3 metres away
12. Small dog behind a wire fence, 1.5 metres away
13. Large dog behind a wire fence, 1.5 metres away
14. Small dog behind a wire fence, 60 cm away
15. Large dog behind a wire fence, 60 cm away
16. Small dog on a lead 18 metres away
17. Large dog on a lead 18 metres away
18. Small dog on a lead 9 metres away

19. Large dog on a lead 9 metres away
20. Small dog on a lead 4.5 metres away
21. Large dog on a lead 4.5 metres away
22. Small dog on a lead 3 metres away
23. Large dog on a lead 3 metres away
24. Small dog on a lead 2 metres away
25. Large dog on a lead 2 metres away
26. Small dog on a lead 1 metre away
27. Large dog on a lead 1 metre away
28. = No. 16 without lead, 29 = No. 17 without lead, and so on, through to No. 39
40. Andy pats small dog
41. Andy pats large dog

The list is a long one, and goes in small steps (they could, if necessary, have been made even smaller, by, for instance, using a medium-sized dog as well, or by using first very short and then gradually longer times for Andy to see or be in company with the dog). It is also pretty complicated (the programme was carried out in a special children's clinic) and some of the steps might be impossible to arrange in a normal situation. This need not matter. The important thing to remember is to make the steps as small as we reasonably can so that moving from one to the next will not be frightening for the child.

When we have made out our hierarchy, we take the first item on it and we present it to the child. If she seems worried by it we stop right there – it shows we haven't gone down far enough in the hierarchy. If she seems completely unconcerned we go to the next step up in the hierarchy and present her with that; and so on until we see the faintest tinge of uneasiness in her. At that point we start the treatment.

Treatment consists of presenting the child with the first item in her hierarchy – the thing that makes her only just anxious – and making the situation, complete with the just-feared thing in it, a pleasant, rewarding, enjoyable one for her; until she loses even that tiny twinge of anxiety. After a while we should be able to present this item to her without her showing the slightest distress. Then we move up to the next step in the hierarchy and repeat the process; presenting the next item to her and making the situation a relaxed, happy one for her. So we gradually work up the hierarchy, until eventually she is no more afraid of that thing than anybody else would be in the same circumstances.

For Andy this meant getting him to the point where he was quite happy in the company of even large friendly dogs. He was not expected to be unafraid of nearby barking dogs – many adults would be afraid in that situation, and quite right too. But Andy was no longer sent running and terrified from harmless dogs, and his life became that much more peaceful and manageable.

The way this treatment works is thought to be something like this. A child with a phobia is afraid of something that is not actually dangerous. She is so afraid of it that she always runs away from it or in some other way avoids it. So she never actually experiences the thing that she fears, so she never learns that it will not hurt her. In graded practice we do two things: present the child with something that is only slightly frightening to her, so that she does not very much want to run away; and we make the situation such a pleasant one that she does not want to run away at all. So she stays in the situation, with the (just-) frightening thing, and she finds she comes to no harm. She stops being afraid of the slightly frightening thing, and we may then go on to repeat the process with the next item up in the hierarchy.

Let us look at an example in detail. Dino had lost most of the use of his legs following an attack of polio and moved about only in a wheelchair. It was thought that he could probably learn to walk with crutches if he wore calipers to support his legs. However, Dino, with a history of a broken leg and some painful experiences in hospital, was terrified of having his legs touched and flew into a screaming tantrum if anyone attempted to do so. It was impossible to measure him for calipers, let alone get him to wear them. So Dino stayed in a wheelchair, until the psychologist working with him decided to try graded practice to get him to allow people to handle and move his legs.

She constructed a hierarchy: the first item was a brief touch of his hand and hand games, working up to the highest items – holding and moving his feet or legs.

The sessions were run as games, since Dino enjoyed these and found them relaxing. First the psychologist modelled the response: she got someone to touch her hand, and showed that this did not frighten her.

'That didn't hurt at all! That was just a touch. Touches don't hurt, Dino. Look, you try it.'

She touched Dino's hand. 'That didn't hurt did it?'

Dino was quite untroubled by this low-on-the-hierarchy item: 'No that didn't hurt.'

'Well *done*, Dino, that was magnificent. You are a very sensible boy.'

Gradually the psychologist progressed from touching Dino's hands and arms to touching his body, then his legs. After eight sessions he would allow his legs to be touched and moved. Things looked good so another attempt was made to put calipers on. Dino reacted with panic, screaming and lashing out uncontrollably. The psychologist realized she had tried to go too fast and that fitting and wearing calipers had to be included in the hierarchy. She went straight back to graded practice and the next few sessions were spent going over the steps in the hierarchy that Dino had already mastered. Then another hierarchy was drawn up, starting with touching Dino's legs with things quite different from calipers (a pencil, an ashtray) then with string, bandages and straps: then all of these were laid one at a time across his legs, then the strings and straps were tied loosely, then done up firmly round his legs. Small parts of the calipers were brought in, and built onto gradually until he was able to put up with complete 'practice calipers'. During this time he had been measured up for his real calipers and in his eighteenth session he put on his own boots for the first time and in the twenty-second allowed the calipers to be strapped on properly. Dino felt enormously proud and excited, and delighted with the praise and pleasure of everyone around him. The whole process had taken four months.

The programme had not gone at all smoothly. Dino was a difficult, touchy, anxious and aggressive boy, and often the psychologist had to wait quietly for him to stop shouting and flailing about, and then go back again to previous steps to allow him to work up slowly to and beyond the point where he had thrown his tantrum. But her patience and persistence resulted in success, and what success! Dino came of a proud Sikh family, who had felt humiliated by having a crippled son who could not walk. When, after weeks of practice with parallel bars and walking frames, he showed them that he could walk his status in the family rose almost visibly. On his thirteenth birthday, twenty months after the treatment was begun, he was given the much-coveted turban that marked his acceptance as an adult Sikh, and which it had once seemed impossible for him ever to attain.

A little girl, Claire, at the age of $2\frac{1}{2}$ developed an intense fear of her own shoes.* It is said of normal adults that when they develop a phobia it is of something potentially dangerous, 'snakes or spiders, but not pyjamas'. But the child with a learning disability may well become phobic about something entirely harmless, as did Claire. She refused to wear shoes, and screamed if she even saw child-sized shoes, though she was not worried by adult-sized shoes. Eventually her parents decided to try graded practice.

Claire was very fond of boiled eggs, and always had one for her tea, so her parents felt that teatime was likely to be a very

---

* The way that Claire's fear was dealt with is described briefly by Lorna Wing, in *Autistic Children: A Guide for Parents* (see Appendix 3). With the author's permission all the steps that were actually followed in helping Claire to overcome her fears are described here.

relaxed, enjoyable time for Claire. They bought a pair of soft slippers in Claire's favourite shade of blue. When Claire was next having a boiled egg they brought the slippers into the room until Claire could just see them; then they took them away again. Claire had shown no sign of distress and continued to eat her egg. The next time, her parents kept the slippers in the room for a little longer while Claire ate her egg; later they were able to bring the slippers gradually nearer and nearer, until they were right beside her chair. On another day, while she was eating her egg they put one slipper on Claire's foot, and took it quickly off again. Later they were able to leave the slipper on for longer, later still to put on the other one. In time she was quite happy to wear the slippers for the whole of teatime. Then, greatly daring, they stood her down on the floor in her slippers – and quickly popped in a mouthful of egg that they had reserved for this moment. After this Claire ran about everywhere in her slippers. Then one day, while she was eating her egg, her father took off one slipper and put on a shoe. No problem. Later in the week the same was done with the other shoe. After this Claire wore shoes like everyone else and as though she had always worn them.

This programme, as it happened, ran smoothly, without hitches or drawbacks. But it might not have done. If a difficulty had arisen her parents would have gone back, as Dino's psychologist did, and repeated the last few successful steps of the hierarchy: then, at the point where trouble had come, they would have put extra steps in the hierarchy so as to take things more slowly. For instance, after getting to the point where she was running round in the slippers Claire might have found the change to shoes on her feet too sudden and too frightening: then her parents would have gone right back to introducing the shoes very gradually into the room, as they had done with the slippers.

Flooding

Sometimes it is just not possible to use graded practice to deal
with a child's fears. It may be that there simply isn't time for
the lengthy process of graded practice to take place, in which
case another possible method to use is flooding. This method
works not by gradually working up to the feared situation but
by presenting the feared situation straight away, in all its most
nerve-wracking aspects – and not allowing the child to get out
of, or avoid the situation.

The reasoning behind this treatment goes like this: as before,
the child is afraid of something that is not dangerous; she
therefore never learns that what she fears is harmless, because
she never gives herself time to experience it. Her getting out of
the feared situation may actually reinforce – strengthen – her
fear: she may think that only her escaping ensures her safety
and she never gives herself the chance to find out that if she
did not escape, if she stayed in the situation, she would come
to no harm.

So in using flooding the child is in some way forced to
remain in the feared situation; and if it is humanly possible,
she is forced to stay in it until she calms down and is no longer
afraid (but see pages 191–2).

How this is done depends on the child and what she is afraid
of. Simon who refused to use any toilet but that in his own
home (see page 74) was made to sit on different toilets: he was
physically held down until he stopped squirming and complaining, accepted them as tolerable and finally used them. A big
moment for Simon's family came when they took him for the
day to the seaside and he used a seaside toilet!

When Claire (see page 186) was older she would, apparently
without any reason, go into screaming panics. Eventually her
parents discovered that this happened when she got damp,
even if it were only a tiny spot of damp on her cuff. At first
they took every possible precaution against her getting this
damp spot; they kept her away from ponds, wash-basins, water
jugs and garden sprinklers, and put an umbrella over her even

before the rain began to fall. If her cuff got wet they changed her dress immediately. At last they saw that life could not go on like this. They altered their tactics. They allowed Claire's cuff to become damp and they held her firmly, not allowing her to throw herself on the ground to rub off the damp or to rip off her cuff, and made her stay put with her damp cuff. After many sessions like this Claire seemed to realize that a damp cuff was not a sign of impending disaster. In time she made no more fuss over it than anyone else would.

Flooding does work in many cases, and it can be quicker than using graded practice. But it is also often hair-raising, as the child may become frantic with terror before she finally calms down, and this can be a very distressing time, especially for her parents. So graded practice is the treatment of choice for phobias. It is calmer, gentler, less fraught for everybody. Probably most of us would prefer to use it whenever possible. But if graded practice is not possible for any reason then it is worth considering using flooding.

Modelling

I mentioned that Dino's psychologist 'modelled' being unafraid of having her hand touched (see page 185). Modelling is a useful extra technique to use along with either graded practice or with flooding. In either case some other person models for the child the unafraid behaviour we want her to show, and this may help her to show it herself. As with modelling in other situations it may be most effective if the person doing the modelling is someone the child is fond of, or someone like herself, like another child (see page 72).

Obsessions

Obsessions are closely related to phobias. Instead of avoiding something, a child with an obsession seems to feel compelled to do something, to carry out some action. People who have obsessions sometimes say they have an indefinable feeling that disaster will strike unless they carry out their rituals – continual hand-washing, going back repeatedly to turn off gas taps or to shut doors, or other kinds of ritual.

Since learning-disabled children with obsessions behave in a very similar way to adult obsessionals, it can be assumed that their reasons for their rituals are much the same. Adults or children, the treatment is to prevent them carrying out their obsessive rituals, and in time they learn that this does not lead to disaster. This technique is rather similar to flooding, in which the phobic person learns that experiencing something, and not avoiding it, does not lead to disaster.

Matthew was 13 years old, a tall handsome boy whose mother had had german measles early in her pregnancy. Matthew had a severe learning disability, was partially deaf, could not speak and had many of the disabilities of a child with autism, amongst them obsessional behaviours. He insisted on certain things being exactly as he wanted them, and always exactly the same. The windows in his house could not be fully opened or closed but had to be opened about three inches, exactly the same amount always all round the house. If the family went for a walk they had always to go along the same route. When they sat together in the evening every member of the family had to sit upright, knees together and heads turned slightly to the right – they were not allowed to cross their legs, or speak or read a paper. If anyone attempted to do something contrary to his obsessions Matthew would throw terrible temper tantrums. He had smashed up most of the home – light fittings, armchairs, TV, the fridge – and the family were very afraid, if they frustrated him, of his attacking his four-year-old sister, the family dog, and little children living nearby. At this point, when the family were spending every evening unable to read, speak or move, they asked for help.

To begin with Matthew went into the local small unit for children with learning disabilities. The staff there got to know him and how to handle him. Because he was in new surroundings he did not show all his old obsessions, but he would still throw tantrums when he did not want to do something. The staff of the unit found that if he was dealt with quietly and firmly and was not allowed to get out of whatever he was supposed to do he would calm down and behave reasonably. His mother, and later his two sisters and his father, visited and were able to work with him in the neutral surroundings of the unit.

Then came the day for Matthew to pay a visit home. He was accompanied by his teacher and psychologist. As soon as he went into the sitting-room of his home, Matthew made a dive at the window, which was shut, and struggled to open it to his required degree. The psychologist retrieved him before he could do so and brought him to sit on the sofa. Matthew threw himself sideways, screamed and tried to bite the psychologist. She made him sit up. Again and again he tried to get to the window, screaming and sobbing, flailing and biting. The psychologist and teacher decided that if he would sit quietly for five minutes they would call it a day. He never did. At the end of an hour he was still fighting and kicking. His parents and sisters were in tears. For practical reasons it was impossible to stay any longer so the psychologist and teacher took him out to the car and back to the unit, convinced that the visit had been a total failure.

Matthew was taken home again the following week. He did not attempt to touch the windows. This time the visit passed in peace, smiles, and congratulations on all sides, especially for Matthew. Nobody was more astonished at the rapidity of the change in Matthew than the psychologist. Like the teacher, she had thought the previous visit had been a disaster, while in any case many treatment programmes of this sort take considerably longer to take effect. It may be, however, that the work that had gone on in the special unit, where Matthew had never been allowed to give free rein to his obsessions, had paved the way for what was an unexpected but most welcome result.

Soon after this Matthew returned home to live. By now his family knew how to manage him. When he tried to impose one of his obsessional rituals they simply did not let him do so – and this included not letting him hurt people around him or damage the house. They had learnt that if they refused to allow him to do these things Matthew, after a period of storms (which became shorter and shorter as time went on), seemed to lose the urge to do them and this gave his family the courage to be firm. They went on a variety of walks around the neighbourhood, and in the evening could read their papers, cross their legs, and talk to each other if they wanted to. Matthew the Tyrant reverted to being Matthew the much-loved son and brother.

Since Matthew could not talk it was impossible to learn what had been going on in his head on that traumatic morning and after, so we can only guess that he had had some vague feeling that something terrible would happen if the window was not opened the required three inches; that he desperately tried to get it open to avert the catastrophe; that when he did not get it open and realized that the catastrophe did not occur he no longer felt it necessary to have the window at that precise angle. This may be a far too simple, or a far too complicated, explanation for Matthew's behaviour, but it is the nearest we can get.

Obsessional objects

Sometimes a child's obsessions take the form of her refusing to be parted from a particular object. Many small children go through a phase of this sort (like Linus in *Peanuts* with his blanket); it may be somewhat inconvenient to the child's parents but not impossibly so, and sooner or later the child herself loses interest in the object and discards it. But a child with a learning disability may become so obsessed with her object that she will not put it down even for a moment, and because her hands are fully occupied with it, cannot learn to do other things like feeding herself or playing with toys.

One way to deal with an obsessional object is similar to graded practice – we gradually reduce its size until it disappears. Peter's object was a blanket, and Claire's an old X-ray film that she had managed to get hold of. In each case their parents snipped a tiny piece off each day until Peter had just a few threads of blanket and Claire a tiny square of X-ray film which she kept tucked in the palm of her hand. Eventually even these fragments disappeared and the children were free to do other things with their hands.

If the obsessional object is something that cannot be so easily cut down, like a toy fire-engine or a watering-can, it may be possible to persuade the child to part from it for increasing lengths of time: first for just a second or two, then ten seconds, half a minute and so on. Ideally the period for which it is taken away will at first be so short that the child will not have time to get upset. If, however, in spite of our efforts she does get upset we have to be very calm and firm and ignore the screams and the tantrums; after a second or two we return the object, and after a rest repeat the process until the child realizes that if she loses her beloved object she soon gets it back again. Then when she is quite calm about losing it for a second or two we can very gradually increase the time, perhaps introducing some other interesting toy or activity while the object is out of the way. The child may in the end learn to do without the object altogether, but if she only learns to do without it for short periods, like half an hour, at least in those times she can do something else with her hands. Timmy, who at first would not be separated from his 'twiddler', learnt to put it down while he was having his meals (see page 33). In time he learnt to put it down when he left the house; after that he spent all day at school without it, which made him a great deal easier to teach.

Better to prevent than cure

Many of the problems that I have been describing are not tackled until they have existed for some time, and this probably makes them more difficult to deal with. The reason they are not dealt with earlier is that at first they may not seem particularly important, and then when they are more pronounced the parents feel forced to accommodate them, allowing the child to keep away from whatever it is she is frightened of. In many cases they do this because the child's reaction is so violent, and they want to avoid this terrible upset. Claire's parents, when they found she was frightened of getting even a tiny spot of water on her, would go to any lengths to circumvent this; and Matthew's family gave in to all his demands because they were so afraid of what he would do if they did not. Although this strategy enabled families to bypass the storms at the time, it did not solve the problem, and in fact the children's demands became more excessive and their own lives more restricted.

So as a general rule, it is best to take action at the first sign of this kind of difficulty, if necessary with the help of the local Community Team for people with learning disabilities or of a local psychologist.

The main points

1. A phobia is a fear which is much greater than the dangerousness of the thing feared warrants.

2. The usual way to treat phobias is by graded practice.

3. The first step is to draw up a hierarchy – a graded scale – of the feared thing.

4. The hierarchy goes from the hardly frightening aspect of the thing to the most frightening that the child needs to cope with.

5. Treatment starts by presenting the first item in the hierarchy when the child is in a pleasant situation.

6. When she shows no concern at the first item we move up to the next item; and so on.

7. In flooding, the child is prevented from escaping from the feared situation.

8. Modelling – someone else demonstrates not being frightened in the feared situation.

9. An obsession is an overwhelming and repeated urge to do some unnecessary action. Response prevention may be used to treat obsessions.

10. Obsessional objects may be either gradually cut down or removed for increasingly long periods.

Some practice problems

*1. Linda has many fears. She is afraid of cats, of very high places (6 metres or more), and of getting dirt on her hands. Her family live in a bungalow and have a poodle as the family pet. She goes to a small village school and her classroom is on the upper floor. Supposing you could treat her fears only one at a time, what order should you take them in?

*2. Bill is terrified of spiders. He does not mind photographs but films of moving spiders make his flesh creep a bit. Can you draw up the possible first (least frightening) six items in his hierarchy?

At the beginning of this book I suggested that, while some people might read it from general interest, others might want to make use of it to help and teach their children. So you may have set up projects to teach putting on a jumper, washing hands, eating with a knife and fork, using signs. In the first flush of enthusiasm perhaps you worked very hard, kept records, perhaps got some surprising and gratifying results. But first enthusiasms simmer down; it may be hard to see how to keep up this level of effort for long. This chapter is written for you: a few ideas to help you carry on.

I'll start with the bugbear of:

Record-keeping

Keeping records is one of the more arduous aspects of working with behavioural methods, and yet it is valuable. By our records we can see progress when otherwise it might be over-looked, spot particular things happening in particular situations (Joe throws most of his temper tantrums after tea and before he goes to bed; Jane can do up buttons below but not above her waist); we can see when our efforts are clearly not having the effect we want and can try something else. Records do help.

So don't abandon record-keeping. However, you probably can lighten the load a bit, particularly when everything is going pretty well. What I am suggesting is that once your programme is under way, don't record everything; instead, record what happens every fourth or seventh or tenth session, or at whatever regular intervals you choose. For instance, if you were teaching Melanie spoon-feeding you could carry out the teaching at every meal (or at every breakfast, or whatever you had decided) but record how many spoonfuls she fed herself, how much prompting she needed, and so on, only on, say, Thursdays. If you were trying to increase the number of times Valerie obeyed verbal requests you might want to have separate records for weekdays and weekends (since she is likely to be given many more requests at weekends, and because the weekend situation is so different from the week, with Dad around more of the time and other people coming and going a good deal). So you might keep records for Sundays and Wednesdays, or Sunday afternoon, or two hours on Sunday, and Wednesday morning before school, whatever seemed suitable to you. The important thing is to keep careful records of everything that happens in the times you have chosen; much better this than recording half of what happens for most of the day. Of course, if what you are recording is something that happens only occasionally – say, heaving flowerpots through a window, or offering to wash up – there is nothing to stop you continuing to record these every time they happen: if you tried to record them in selected short periods you might never catch them.

Keeping regular, but not continuous, records like this makes record-keeping less of a drag and perhaps more practicable in the long run. There are just a few things to watch out for.

First, try to ensure as far as you can that the time you pick for your recordings is a fairly typical one. For instance, we would not choose to record Valerie's obedience the day that an aunt, who doesn't think it fair to be hard on the child and does everything for her, regularly comes to tea. If the aunt happened to come to tea on the day set aside for recording obedience, we would note that the day was an unusual one and would go ahead with our recording. Similarly, if Melanie's favourite food was ice-cream, we would not have ice-cream *always* on Thursdays: ice-cream would be on the menu sometimes on Thursdays, sometimes on other days. Make sure, too, that the length of time for which you make your recordings stays the same: you don't want to try to compare the number of toileting successes per day before treatment with the number of toileting successes per half day afterwards.

Second, we should try to make sure that the teaching continues, and that we put as much effort into it, on the days when we were not making recordings as on the days when we are. One of the spin-offs of record-keeping is that it does seem to make the work more worthwhile: just because we are easing the burden of recording for ourselves we don't want the work itself to fall off.

Third, as I hinted earlier, these discontinuous but regular records are adequate and practical when everything is going along well. If you hit a difficult patch, it may be helpful to go back to keeping fuller, continuous records, because they are more likely to tell you what is going wrong. Do you have more difficulty on certain days? When certain people are around? Or not around? When your child is more likely to be tried? Or when she has been involved in certain activities? When she is in certain places? And so on. You are more likely to get this sort of information from continuous records, and so be able to see what changes you could make in your programme.

To sum up: record-keeping can be wearisome (I am smitten to the heart by the memory of someone saying to me, '*Please* can we have a break over Christmas?' and feel sure that, at least in part, a break was needed from record-keeping) but it is worthwhile and rewarding. Find a reasonably typical time, at whatever regular interval seems to you appropriate, and keep records only then. If you run into difficulties with your programme it may be worth going back to keeping more continuous records.

Of course, if what is driving you mad is the pressure of carrying out the teaching sessions themselves, then you should consider spacing them out a bit – mad parents are unlikely to be a great help to the child. However, spacing out the teaching may slow up the child's learning, whereas spacing out recordings should not. So, if you decide to space out the teaching sessions, you should be prepared for the child to learn rather more slowly.

What to do when you are stuck

It is easy enough to carry out programmes when everything is going swimmingly. It is not so easy when things go wrong, the programme doesn't seem to work, the child stops progressing. What then? I certainly do not have all the answers but here are a few tips that may help.

1. *Examine the problem*

Look as closely as you can at what has been happening. Look at the methods you have used to try to solve the problem: if they have failed, try to see the possible reasons for their failure – every reason you can think of, not just the most obvious or probable. Work out as clearly as you can what the difficulty is. Write it down.

At this point you are not trying to find solutions, just to get a clear picture of the problem.

2. *Discuss it*

Two heads are better than one. It is a lonely business trying to grapple with difficulties in a programme on your own. Try, however, to discuss it with somebody who has some knowledge of and interest in behavioural methods or you may find yourselves at cross purposes – common sense is not quite the same. Other parents who have been trying to use these methods may be willing to help, and may in their turn enlist your help with their problems. You might also get in touch with the divisional general manager of MENCAP, or with a local psychologist, if necessary via the British Psychological Society (see Appendix 2).

3. *Solutions*

Once you are quite clear what the problem is, possible solutions often (though not always) become more obvious. For example, when Jack was learning to put on his socks he got stuck at the stage where he had to pull the sock over his heel (see page 115). It wasn't until his teacher saw that the difficulty lay in the position Jack sat in, with his heel resting across the other knee, that she realized he needed to have his foot free of contact. Even so her first solution – to get Jack to put his foot on the floor – failed; after that she gave him a chair to rest his foot on and Jack quickly learnt to pull on his socks.

Sometimes the best way to deal with a problem may not be to tackle it directly but to try to deal with it by working on something else. With children who are aggressive, instead of trying to stop the behaviour we may try to lessen its frequency by encouraging – reinforcing – other, better things. Or again, we may look to see whether a simple change in the child's surroundings – a higher chair at the table, a gate to keep her out of the kitchen, an electric night-light, a zip instead of buttons, a lock on the china cupboard – can help to change her behaviour in the direction we want it to go. These two methods are, of course, DRO (Differential Reinforcement of Other kinds of behaviour) and changing the surroundings, which are discussed in chapter 7, 'Learning not to'. Because they are indirect ways of tackling a problem they are easy to overlook. It is worth keeping them in mind, especially when more direct methods don't seem to be working.

I suggested on page 66, that if a programme stopped working there were two questions you should ask yourself. First, are the reinforcers really effective? And, second, has the task been broken down into small enough steps? Whether the second applies will depend on what you are working on (it probably would not apply if, for instance, you were trying to deal with tantrums) but the first may always apply. It is extremely common for a child to lose interest in a reinforcer, and you should not be discouraged if she goes right off something on which until recently her whole happiness apparently depended. It is then important to look for what *is* now reinforcing to her and not to think 'reinforcers don't work'. It is a question of

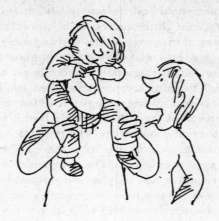

finding the right one. With some children this can be very, very difficult; but it is crucial to what we do.

Finally, three points. It is always worth asking yourself whether you have been consistent in carrying out the treatment. When people say, as they often do, 'We've tried everything', they may well have gone through many of the approaches that I have described but in a rather half-hearted fashion. Perhaps because they were not entirely convinced that they were doing the best thing, they used the treatment at some times but not others. So, without castigating yourself for backsliding, in future try to be consistent; then you can decide whether it is or it isn't the best thing to do.

Secondly, when you are considering possible solutions to your problem, try to be flexible and to keep an open mind. Obviously you have to choose the most likely solution but it may help if you define clearly *why* one is more likely to succeed than another; in particular when everything seems unlikely it may be necessary to stop saying, '*That* won't work', and give it a try. In any case you will need to keep careful records of what you do, and, probably, set a time limit for how long you will try it.

This brings me to the last point: a programme must be given time to work, and should not be said to have failed until it has been going long enough for success to be possible. One of the repeated findings of many researches is that people with learning disabilities *can* learn, and often do learn, to do tasks as well as anybody else, but it takes them much longer to reach the same standard. The crunch comes when you ask, how long is long enough? There is no general answer to that question – the answer will depend on the task, the child, how often you have your teaching sessions, and so on. The important thing is not to give up almost as soon as you have started. Over and over again I have heard people say, 'The programme's no good, it isn't working' – and it was only agreed on yesterday. It may help if, when you set out on a programme, you decide on a period of time for which you will keep it up – say, a week, or ten days, or twelve teaching sessions. At the end of that time, but not before, unless disaster strikes (and not counting small adjustments to the programme) you will look at it again, and decide whether to carry on or whether to change the programme. You don't want to struggle on indefinitely with something that is clearly not useful, but neither do you want to abandon a promising programme before it has had a chance to succeed.

The following check-list may help you to pinpoint problems.

1. *Reinforcement*

If social (praise, hugs, etc.): are these really enthusiastic and clear?

If edible (sweets, fruit, cheese, drinks, etc.): has she got tired of it? (Try something else.)

Is the rate of reinforcement right (i.e. is it given often enough)?

Does she get the reinforcement too freely at other times (e.g. biscuits for elevenses and tea *and* for her teaching sessions)?

Is the reinforcement given quickly enough (immediately after the good behaviour)?

Would a different reinforcer help (e.g. a favourite toy instead of a sweet, a lick on a lolly to back up the 'good girl')?

2. *Teaching new skills*

Has the task been broken down into small enough steps?

Is enough physical prompting being given?

Have the prompts been faded out too quickly? Not enough?

Is the child gradually doing a little more, and then a little more still, for each reinforcer?

Is the task one that the child is really likely to be able to succeed in, or is it a bit too ambitious? It is not always easy to tell in advance what it will or will not be possible to teach to a particular child, and sometimes we just have to go ahead and try teaching it to her (see pages 58–9). But if after a spell of careful teaching, and if none of the suggestions in this section make a difference, it may be better to go back to an easier task and work up, or to leave this task for a while and return to it later.

Is the child bored? (Although this is usually because she is no longer interested in the reinforcer, it can be that she is bored with the task.)

Are the sessions the right length (i.e. not too long)?

Would it be better to have shorter, more frequent sessions?

3. *Bad behaviour*

Are you sure the 'bad' behaviour is not still being reinforced (e.g. by a brother/sister/uncle/teacher)?

Are you quite clear what is the reinforcer for the 'bad' behaviour?

Very important: If her 'bad' behaviour is no longer being reinforced, does the child get plenty of reinforcement for her good behaviour instead?

If absolutely desperate: try rereading chapters 3 to 7. See if this suggests anything that you haven't already used, try it boldly, keeping careful records of what happens.

To encourage the others

You may find that you have been able to achieve quite considerable changes with your child. A persistent wetter may have become toilet-trained, an uncooperative child more amenable, a child with limited skills able to do more for herself. If you feel that what you have done would be of interest or benefit to other parents, think about writing a short account of it for publication, either in your local newsletter, or in *Parents' Voice*, or in one of the journals. Your local psychologist or MENCAP representative should be able to give help if you want it. Nothing succeeds like success, and I can imagine few things more encouraging to parents than to hear what other parents, through their own initiative and effort, have been able to do for their own children.

Good luck!

Appendixes

Appendix 1: Answers to the Practice Problems

These are some answers I can suggest to the 'practice problems' marked with an asterisk in the text.

Chapter 3: Reinforcement

4. Housework, for example; it must be one of the most under-reinforced of all activities. I bet you can count on the fingers of one hand the number of times it's even noticed – 'How nicely the bedroom has been dusted' or 'This shirt has been beautifully ironed'. It is lucky we get some satisfaction from the sight of dust-free surfaces and wrinkle-free shirts or we might be unlikely to dust or iron very often.

5. When the child gets the sweet she stops complaining of the pain: her parents experience relief from her complaining and are negatively reinforced – they are more likely to give her a sweet on another occasion. But the child receives a sweet when she complains, so her complaining is positively reinforced: she is likely to complain more often.

   The outcome is likely to be that the child will complain of more and more pains. If her parents realize that what they are doing – giving the sweets – is increasing her complaints they might decide to act differently. They would of course keep a sharp lookout for any genuine illness but if they thought there was nothing the matter with the child (as they clearly did when they 'cured' her with a sweet) they might say pleasantly that little girls with pains shouldn't eat sweets; they might distract her with something to look at or do; and when some time had gone by without her complaining she might then be offered a sweet. If the child found that she never got sweets when she said she had a pain she might complain less.

Chapter 4: Star Charts and Tokens

3. The first move is to check on the exchange reinforcers – are they powerful enough? Is she really keen to get them? If she is carelessly mislaying her tokens it may be that she doesn't much care about them because she doesn't much care about the exchange reinforcers. If we suspect this is the case we should look around for something that she would like very much.

If, however, we think that she *does* care about the exchange reinforcers then we might try to devise some better way for her to store her tokens once they have been given to her: a necklace with a fool-proof clasp, or a string attached to her belt ending in a tag (these two would only work with tokens that have a hole in the middle); or a purse with a flap with a Velcro fastening on a belt. Or the tokens could be put into a rack or jar where she could see them but would not have to carry them about.

4. We should have to use something that was available on the desert island; but it must not be something so easily available that the child (or whoever the programme was for) could pick it up easily and so come into possession of quantities of unearned 'tokens'. So it would have to be something that only we had access to; the tail feathers of our pet parrot who would allow no one else to touch him, or a particular kind of shell, the source of which only we knew. Or we could use something quite commonplace like pebbles or peeled twigs but mark it with something that only we had – the cochineal we happened to have saved from the shipwreck, or the only ball-point pen on the island.

This question obviously has some relevance for real life. The child should not be able to cheat by pretending she has earned more tokens than she really has. So the tokens, or stars or whatever, must be kept carefully out of reach.

5. All sorts of things may contribute to the failure of a slimmer's programme, and I can only suggest a few of them.

Has the slimmer chosen adequate exchange reinforcers? In my own programme I once caught myself thinking, 'Well I don't care about the reinforcer anyway'. I had to change the reinforcer, fast.

Is the reinforcer immediate enough? Especially in the case of slimming. The pleasure to be got from eating is so strong and so immediate that only a very powerful reinforcer, the prospect of which is clearly in front of the slimmer, has a hope of competing with food. For this reason (immediacy of reinforcement) it is probably better too for the tokens to be earned for what is or is not eaten, rather than for weight loss, which is rather far removed from the crucial factor of eating. The effect might be even greater if tokens were also earned for *not buying* the food.

Does the slimmer have a reasonable hope of getting the reinforcement? Or is the programme too stringent? If hopelessness has set in it may be better to relax the rules slightly and then build up gradually.

If penalties are incurred for failure, are these too severe? Again, this happened in my programme, when the penalty (not having a bath) was so unpleasant that I kept letting myself off. The programme worked better when I fixed on something (no orange juice for breakfast) that, though I disliked it, I was prepared to impose on myself.

If the programme is entirely self-controlled it could be beneficial to enlist the help of someone else to monitor successes and failures. Having to confess to my family that I had not earned my orange juice made me more likely to ensure that I did earn it.

Family support may be especially important for the slimmer. She (or he) needs her family to back her up, to urge her on, to encourage rather than deride or to undermine the programme as one kind-hearted but misguided husband did, who gave his wife a large box of chocolates because he felt so sorry for her.

6. There are several things we could do.

(*a*) If he was very slow we might gradually speed up Charlie's dressing by requiring him to do it in a shorter time. At first he might have no time limit at all, then to earn the tokens he might have to get dressed within forty-five minutes, then forty minutes, and so on until he was dressing within a reasonable time.

(*b*) We could extend the things he needed to do to earn the sweets – washing himself, or helping to lay the table.

Neither of these would reduce the number of sweets he got. If we thought it *very* important to do that we could:

(*c*) Reduce the number of tokens he earned, and tell him, first, that he would now get one token for the pair of socks; then, when he was used to that, that he would get one token for vest and pants; and so on; *or*,

(*d*) Increase the 'token price' of the sweets; we could tell him that three tokens were needed now for two sweets; *or*,

(*e*) Include other kinds of reinforcers that he could exchange for his tokens: some special treat for breakfast, five minutes cuddling, five minutes with a tape-recorder – anything we could think of that he would like as an alternative to the sweets.

Chapter 5: Teaching by Guiding

4. (*a*) We would make her hook much bigger than those of the rest of the family, so that it stood out and was more obvious. This would make it more likely that she would have little difficulty in picking it out as hers, even if at first she needed some prompting to go to it. When she was confidently and regularly hanging her coat on it we would make the hook a little smaller; later a little smaller still, and so on. Eventually she should be able to go straight to her own peg even when it was similar to everyone else's.

(*b*) We would start by giving her large buttons and large

buttonholes to work on, perhaps on a pyjama top. Later, as she became skilful with these, we could give her a series of smaller buttons and holes.

(c) We would make the word 'Tea' particularly arresting, either by making the letters bigger than the letters for 'Sugar' or 'Rice' or by giving them a vivid outline or backing, say in bright red. As she became able to pick out the canister we would fade this, either by making the letters gradually smaller or by fading the colour to a paler red, then to pink, and later to nothing.

Later on of course we might do the same thing for the other canisters.

(d) We would give her fairly firm (quite thick) slices of bread and nicely softened butter to work with.

It's all pretty obvious really, but it does help.

Chapter 6: Imitation: Learning by Copying

1. Most sports – tennis, golf, football – are taught very largely through imitation, though occasionally a teacher will use a certain amount of prompting especially on hand and arm movements.

Here are a few more:
Singing
Dancing
Plaiting
Stirring and beating in cookery.

Can you think of others?

2. Prompting could be used, but would be clumsy and tedious. Most could be done to a certain extent by following instructions, either verbal or written; but imitation is a much easier and surer way to teach.

3. Sleeping in a bed.

Sometimes children who are used to sleeping in their own bed will not sleep if they go in a strange bed. Usually they accept the new bed after a night or two, or they may be helped by bringing some familiar things from the old bed – their teddy-bear, a special pillow or blanket.

5. (*a*) Rain falling. A wet weather forecast. Seeing other people in mackintoshes or with umbrellas. A threatening sky.
(*b*) Traffic already on the road. Road signs (*Tenez la droite*).
(*c*) Somebody wearing a deaf aid. Noisy surroundings. Somebody not replying, or saying 'Eh?' when we speak in a normal voice. Somebody at a distance.
(*d*) Seeing a charity flag seller. A request – 'That will be 50p'. Being given a bill. A ring on the front door bell following a muffled rendition of the first verse of 'Oh come all ye faithful'.
(*e*) An alarm clock going off. A baby crying. Hearing other people about. A full bladder. Somebody shaking you or saying 'Get up'. A smell of fire.

Chapter 7: Learning Not To

1. Either you would have to arrange to meet your *bête noire* personally or, if he/she were going to appear in public, you would have to organize the entire audience to carry out the treatment. You would also have to find out what was the reinforcer maintaining the *bête noire*'s 'bad' behaviour, but I think we can expect that in most of these cases it is applause. Then, whether in private or public meetings, if you are using extinction (*a*), when the 'bad' behaviour appeared it would be met by blank silence. Similarly if you were using time-out (*b*), the *bête noire* would receive a good deal of applause which would stop abruptly when he produced the 'bad' behaviour.

2. (*a*) Extinction and DRO. We would expect that attention

is the reinforcer. We would look rather uninterested in the stories of her illnesses but become immediately interested if she talked about anything else. We might also prompt her to show the kind of behaviour that would be reinforced by leading the conversation on to other topics – such as how she grew the fruit and flowers, and how good she was at this.

(b) First, we would consider the surroundings. Have the boys adequate facilities in which to hang up or otherwise store their clothes? Yes, of course they have. All right then (but I once revolutionized my own willingness to put books away properly by reorganizing things so that the books would actually go into the bookshelves). Next, having decided against threatening them with draconian penalties ('No pocket-money for a month if I ever see any garment of yours on the floor'), it is back to reinforcing the desired behaviour. We contract to give the boys something they would like each time an evening inspection shows the floor clear of clothing (which has not been just bundled under the bed). If what they want is something fairly major we would negotiate a token system – a ticket for a concert for twenty-eight clear-floor evenings, for example. If this went well we would negotiate another, aiming to stretch the reinforcement a bit, or until the boys said, 'Oh, for heaven's sake, mother, we don't need to go on with this, we take your point' – by now they have come to find it just as easy and rather pleasanter to put their clothes away as it is to drop them on the floor. At least I hope they have.

(c) Extinction. But make sure she has been to the lavatory before you set off for your shopping. And it might be a good idea to make the conversations few and brief, and to hand out reinforcement if she did not interrupt (DRO).

(d) I am really stumped by this one. I think I would put up with it, or try to forestall it by expressing appreciation first. But it does get boring to have to do that for every meal. Has anybody any better ideas?

(*e*) Change the surroundings – put the butter somewhere where he can't get it. And make sure he gets a drop of cream every now and again in his saucer.

Chapter 8: Dressing and Undressing

1. (a) *Mitts*

Adult	Child
1. Puts mitt over child's hand, guides thumb almost in	1. Holds cuff of mitt, pulls mitt fully on
2. Puts mitt over child's hand, guides thumb half-way in	2. Holds cuff, pushes thumb in and pulls mitt fully on
3. Puts mitt over child's hand, guides thumb to thumb hole	3. Holds cuff, pushes thumb right in and pulls mitt fully on
4. Puts mitt over hand	4. Holds cuff, finds thumb hole, pulls mitt on
5. Puts mitt half over hand	5. Pulls mitt on to hand, finding thumb hole
	6. Puts mitt on

 (b) *Woolly hat*

Adult	Child
1. Puts hat on to child's forehead, pulls back and down over ears	1. Pushes front of hat back on forehead
2. Puts hat on to child's forehead, pulls back and down nearly over ears	2. Pulls right down, adjusts front
3. Pulls hat half-way over ears	3. Pulls down and adjusts front
4. Pulls hat to ears	4. Pulls hat out (if she does not do this she is liable to end up with her ears folded down in half) over ears and down, adjusts front
5. Puts hat to forehead	5. Pulls hat down, out, and down and adjusts
	6. Puts hat on

(c) Wellington boots

1. Finds support for child to lean on (wall, back of chair, etc.) lifts one foot, puts it into boot until heel almost down	1. Pushes foot flat and fully into boot
2. Puts foot half-way into foot of boot, heel raised	2. Pushes foot fully into boot
3. Puts foot into boot until toe touches the bottom	3. Slides foot into foot of boot
4. Puts foot half-way into leg of boot	4. Pushes foot down leg and into foot of boot
5. Puts foot into mouth of leg-opening of boot	5. Pushes foot right down leg and into foot of boot
6. Provides support for child	6. Lifts foot, puts it into boot and pushes it fully down
	7. Leans for support, and puts foot into boot

2. (a) Probably (I think) putting in the first arm (steps 8 to 9): otherwise pulling it over her head (step 10) especially if it is a jumper with a close neck, like a polo neck.

(b) Finding the second armhole (step 6). Always the bogey in my experience.

(c) Pushing the (black) lace under the (white) loop, and through to make the second loop (step 3). Everything else is plain sailing compared with this.

3. (a) A woman's one-piece swimsuit: and, perhaps, other garments which are dry when you put them on and wet when you take them off.

(b) Rubber gloves, if you take them off right side out. They are quite easy if you peel them off, like surgeons do, but then you have the bother of putting them right side out again (unless you are a surgeon, I suppose, in which case you leave it to a minion, or just throw the gloves away).

(c) Wellington boots. Especially if they are a bit big they are very easy to slip on, but taking them off entails quite a tricky bit of pressing the toe of one foot against the heel of the other.

Chapter 9: Washing

1. We would concentrate the teaching on the bath, though it would not hurt to repeat things at the wash-basin when he was washing his hands. We would teach him the difference between the hot and cold taps: these would be clearly marked, with a large red (for hot) and blue (for cold) sticker. We would test the water in each, and get Bobby to test it and show him the stickers and emphasize 'Cold', 'Hot'.

Then we would run some water into the bath, rather cool perhaps, test it, and get Bobby to do so: we would say (something like), 'Wants more *hot*' and prompt him to turn on the hot tap. We would keep testing, and getting him to, until the right temperature had been reached: then we would say, 'Enough!' and prompt Bobby to turn off the tap. Then, if he wanted to, he would be allowed to get into the bath and play in it.

We would repeat the process with too hot water and adding cold, being especially careful and only letting Bobby put in a fingertip. Then we would go on to letting Bobby do the testing first, and reinforcing him if he made the right decision, either that the water was a reasonable temperature, or that it needed more of either hot or cold.

Finally, at the end of the teaching process, Bobby would test his bathwater temperature every night, and we would check it until we were quite sure he could be safely left to do it on his own. We wouldn't worry too much if the water was a bit too cool but be very, very careful about its being too hot.

2. For me, there seem to be four ways.

    (*a*) As a routine – on getting up and on going to bed, before meals and after going to the toilet.

    (*b*) If my hands feel sticky.

    (*c*) If I have been handling something dirty or unhygienic.

    (*d*) If I can see dirt on them. How much dirt there needs to be depends on what I am about to do; if I am going to do cooking, or sewing, or handle clothes straight from the washing machine the smallest speck will suffice to send me to the wash-basin; if I am going to garden, or bath the dog, or go for a walk I would not be so fussy.

Chapter 10: Dry Pants, Dry Bed

The child might be frightened of or unhappy on the potty. In this case we would try to make sitting on the potty a happy time for her: we would give her her favourite toys, play or sing with her, perhaps give her little bits of favourite food, in the hope that she would begin to relax enough to use the potty.

Or she might associate wetting so strongly with the feeling of wearing nappies or pants that they have become to her the cue for wetting, and she cannot allow herself to wet when she is not wearing them. We would wait until it was warm enough to let her run about all day without any pants on, and then try again.

Or she may just do it to annoy, in which case we would remain very calm and unperturbed; and we would try sitting her on the pot, getting her off it, then just before the two minutes was up, we would sit her down again. And if by chance she then performed, ply her lavishly with every reinforcer at our command.

Chapter 11: Eating and Table Manners

1. I think this would have to be taught by imitation, with a minimal amount of physical prompting, because the very fine finger adjustments needed would, I think, be very difficult to prompt. If the child was not able to learn by imitation I should gratefully recall that the Chinese use a spoon a good deal and would teach this skill to the child instead.

2. Chips, toast (in fingers if buttered, with knife and fork if under scrambled egg), lettuce, tomato, cucumber, apples, cream cakes, chicken drumsticks.

The cues that tell us whether or not we should use our fingers are quite complicated. They depend partly on the state of the food — hot or cold, dry or a bit messy, as for instance a dressed salad; partly on the situation — a dinner party or a picnic; partly on what other people are doing. This last might be the most useful guide for the child; if we could teach her to see what other people do before she starts to eat she might make fewer mistakes. Otherwise a few simple rules might help: 'It's *hot*, use your knife and fork,' 'We're *in the garden*, you can use your fingers'.

It *is* complicated, so perhaps it is just as well that it does not matter very much.

3. Imitation, and/or prompting, and breaking down the activity into small steps. We could show the child how to put a knife on the right-hand side of one person's place: then at each person's place. Then we could go on to a knife and fork: then knife, fork and plate: and so on.

We could also change the surroundings by putting a large sheet of paper, with knife, fork, spoon, plate and cup drawn on it, at each person's place, and the child would put the objects in their place over the picture of each one. Later we fade this prompt by making the drawings gradually fainter and fainter, while making sure that the child can still succeed at every stage.

4. We would give Lucy a plate on a suction mat (see Appendix 4). We would watch her like a hawk as she reaches the end of the meal. As she went to tip the plate we would prevent her from doing so; and we would prompt her to say, or make a sign, or produce a picture card, for the word 'Finished'. Then we would reinforce her and take her plate away. We would do this at every meal until she found it was no longer necessary to tip her plate.

If, despite our efforts, Lucy managed occasionally to tip her plate over, we would retrieve the plate and make her say or sign that she had finished.

Chapter 12: Play

2. Deaf/blind children can enjoy: Play-doh; Plasticine, sand, water, including baths and swimming; movement – swings, pushcarts, rockers, bouncy cushions; 'feely box' and 'feely toy' – these are not so far as I know available commercially but are quite easy to make. A 'Feely box' consists of a box containing all sorts of things which feel interesting and different from each other – soft, hard, knobbly, smooth, scratchy, silky, furry, round, square, tubular and so on. The box might have, amongst other things, shells, pieces of macaroni, big round beads, square beads, soft woolly balls, small bricks covered with sandpaper and others covered with mock fur. The child can feel about in the box, encountering different and unexpected textures. A 'feely toy' is based on the same idea but the different materials are built onto a board, or stitched onto a doll or a teddy bear – an example of this kind of toy is described in an article by Geraldine McCormack and Mona Tsoi, 'Toys for the multiply handicapped child', *Apex*, Vol. 4, 1976, pp. 24–6.

Blind children may enjoy all these but can also enjoy noise – music-makers – humming tops, rattles, drums, xylophones, hammer toys; squeaky toys.

Sense: The National Deafblind and Rubella Association have an excellent list of toys and activities for deaf/blind children – see Appendix 2.

3. First, we would make sure that there were plenty of things that the child *could* do: outdoor things if possible like a swing, tricycle or bike, slide or climbing-frame; indoor things like jigsaws, building bricks, constructional toys, materials for drawing, painting, colouring, cutting and sticking; picture books and comics; the makings of imaginative play – dressing-up things, dolls, cars and garages, teasets and toy guns. We would make a list of these, using pictures if the child could not read.

Then we would tell her that she would get a little reward, or a star to stick on her chart, every time she came and told us what she was going to do instead of asking what she could do (we might have to set some limit on how often this could be – three times in half an hour perhaps). If she did come and ask we would prompt her to look at her list and decide for herself.

4. We would use graded practice (see chapter 13), prompting and reinforcement. Suppose it is Rex, whom we want to help to play with other children. We would set up a very pleasant situation in which Rex got lots of adult attention. Then we would bring another child, Mark, into the far end of the room. (It helps if Mark is himself a friendly, sociable person.) Gradually over many sessions we would get Mark to draw nearer and nearer to Rex, always making sure that Rex was quite calm and relaxed. When Mark was able to be quite near to Rex we would have him first look, then smile at Rex, then pass him an object, then touch him. We would teach Mark to give social reinforcement to Rex in just the same way as we did: to begin with, Mark could give the reinforcement simultaneously with us – for instance we would smile and stroke Rex's cheek and say, 'Well done, that's *lovely*!' at the same time. Gradually we would fade out our part in the reinforcement so that eventually it was given only by Mark. We would go on to prompt Rex to give an object to Mark, to touch him, to begin to play some simple game that Rex enjoys with him; and keep our warmest reinforcement for the occasions when he does so.

All this is likely to take quite some time and several sessions: we would not expect to get Mark sitting right next to Rex at the first attempt, but would expect to take it very slowly.

Chapter 13: Getting Over Phobias and Obsessions

1. Since Linda does not have to cope with either high places or cats in her daily life the first fear we would tackle is that of getting dirt on her hands. This problem may crop up at any time, and especially if she does painting or cookery, while it could also make it difficult for her to learn to wipe herself at the toilet.

Probably the second fear to tackle would be that of cats, as she could encounter a cat if she visited relatives or her friends. Lastly, we would expect to try to help her to get over her fear of high places.

However, this order could be rearranged if, as we got to know Linda better, we found there were particular reasons to do so – if, for instance, we found that the next-door neighbours had just got a cat that often strayed into Linda's garden. The order in which we would tackle the problems would be that which would give the greatest benefit to Linda.

2.   1. Film of stationary spider (long shot).
   2. Film of stationary spider (close-up).
   3. Spider in film moves one leg.
   4. Spider in film moves one inch.
   5. Spider in film moves three inches.
   6. Spider in film moves across the screen.

We should have to discuss these with Bill or try them out to see whether they were suitable steps, or whether he needed smaller ones. We could go on to toy spiders, toy spiders that move, dead little spiders, dead big ones, small live ones in a confined space and far away from Bill, then coming gradually closer. And so on.

Appendix 2: Useful Addresses

British Epilepsy Association, Anstey House, 40 Hanover Square, Leeds, LS3 1BE. Tel: (Freefone for advice and information) 0800 30 90 30. Provides care in the community for people with epilepsy, and an advice and information service on all aspects of epilepsy.

British Psychological Society, St Andrews House, 48 Princess Road East, Leicester LE1 7DR. Information, and contacts for local psychological services.

Contact a Family, 170 Tottenham Court Road, London W1P 0HA. Tel: 0171 383 3555. Fax: 0171 383 0259. Provides links between families and between families and local or national self-help groups. Good source of information about other specialist groups.

Disabled Living Foundation (DLF), 380–384 Harrow Road, London W9 2HU. Tel: 0171 289 6111 (1–4 pm) (for appointments to view equipment). Fax: 0171 266 2922. Information service, especially regarding equipment for daily living needs (please write).

Down's Syndrome Association, 153–155 Mitcham Road, London SW17 9PG. Tel: 0181 682 4001 (24-hour helpline). Fax: 0181 682 4012. Help and support for children with Down's syndrome and their families.

Makaton Vocabulary Development Project, 31 Firwood Drive, Camberley, Surrey GU15 3QD. Tel: 01276 61390. Fax: 01276 681368. Provides information and guidance on the use of Makaton, and details of training and resource materials, to parents, carers and professionals.

MENCAP (Royal Society for Mentally Handicapped Children and Adults), MENCAP National Centre, 123 Golden Lane, London EC1Y 0RT. Tel: 0171 454 0454. Fax: 0171 608 3254. Provides homes, leisure activities (Gateway clubs), and a range of other services (for example, legal, welfare and benefit advice). The bookshop is the only specialist bookshop in the country and runs a mail-order service.

MIND – National Association for Mental Health, Granta House, 15–19 Broadway, London E15 4BQ. Tel: 0181 519 2122. Fax: 0181 522 1725. Pressure group on behalf of people with any form of mental disorder. Provides services, homes, publications, training, conferences.

National Association of Toy and Leisure Libraries – Play Matters, 68 Churchway, London NW1 1LT. Tel: 0171 387 9592. Fax: 0171 383 2714. Information about and contacts for toy and leisure libraries, provides publications.

National Autistic Society, 276 Willesden Lane, London NW2 5RB. Tel: 0181 451 1114. Fax: 0181 451 5865. Runs schools and adult centres, offers a range of support, advice and information services. Supports the Centre for Social and Communication Disorders, Elliot House, Masons Hill, Bromley, Kent BR2 9HT. Tel: 0181 466 0098. Fax: 1081 466 0118) which offers diagnosis, assessment, professional training and research.

Royal Society for Mentally Handicapped Children and Adults, see MENCAP.

Scope (formerly the Spastics Society), 12 Park Crescent, London W1N 4EQ. Tel: 0171 636 5020. 01800 626216 (Cerebral Palsy help-line, Mon-Fri 11am–9pm, Sat, Sun 2–6 pm). Fax: 0171 436 2601. Services for people with cerebral palsy (including those with learning disabilities): schools, further education and residential care.

Sense: The National Deafblind and Rubella Association, 11–13 Clifton Terrace, London N4 3SR. Tel: 0171 272 7774. Fax: 0171 272 6012. The national voluntary organization which campaigns for the needs of deaf/blind children, providing advice, support, information and services for them, their families and professionals in the field.

Appendix 3: Useful Books

General

Children with Mental Retardation: A Parents' Guide, Romayne Smith (ed.), Woodbine House, 1993. American, very readable, lots of down-to-earth quotes from parents.

Listen to Me: Communicating the Needs of People with Profound Intellectual and Multiple Disabilities, Pat Fitton, Jessica Kingsley Publishers, 1994. Based on the author's experiences with her own severely disabled daughter. Especially good on how to convey a child's needs when away from home, in school, hospital, respite care.

Teaching disabled children

Starting Off: Establishing Play and Communication in the Handicapped Child, Chris Kiernan, Rita Saunders and Chris Jordan, Souvenir Press, London, 1978. Teaching for those with the most severe disabilities.

Let Me Speak, Dorothy M. Jeffree and Roy McConkey, Souvenir Press, London, 1991. Teaching language. Written particularly for parents.

Basic Abilities: a whole approach, Sophie Levitt, Souvenir Press, 1994. How to teach daily living skills, play, movement. Illustrated by the author.

For later on: *Working Towards Independence*, Janet Carr and Suzanne Collins, Jessica Kingsley Publishers, 1992. Similar approach to the present book but written for those working with adults rather than with children with learning disabilities.

Toys and play

Play Helps: Toys and Activities for Children with Special Needs, Roma Lear, Heinemann Medical Books, London, 1980. Full of ideas on toys to buy and to make, and games to play with children with disabilities, grouped according to the senses – 'Making the most of' – sight, hearing, touch and smell. Cheerful text and illustrations. Also: *More Play Helps: Play Ideas for Children with Special Needs*, Roma Lear, Heinemann Medical Books, 1990. Alphabetical guide to DIY toys and activities, from suggestions sent in by parents, teachers, etc.

Let Me Play, Dorothy Jeffree, Roy McConkey and Simon Hewson, Souvenir Press, London, 1988. Lots of ideas on helping a child to play, and making and using special toys for a disabled child.

Good catalogues from:

Toys for the Handicapped, 76 Barracks Road, Sandy Lane Industrial Estate, Stourport-on-Severn, Worcestershire DY13 9QB. Tel: 01299 827820. Very well-made toys, specially designed for disabled children. Prices rather high for the average family but would be worth clubbing together for.

Early Learning Centre, local branches or from South Marston, Swindon SN3 4TJ. Tel: 01793 831300

Feeding

Helping the Handicapped Child with Early Feeding: a manual for parents and professionals, Jennifer Warner, Winslow Press, 1981. Obtainable, free (while stocks last), on receipt of an A4 envelope with first class stamp, from: Ms J. Warner, Department of Speech Pathology and Therapy, The University, Manchester M13 9PL. Contains sound advice on the best position for feeding, utensils, moving from liquid to solid food, and much else.

Children with particular disabilities

Autism

Autistic Children: A Guide for Parents, Lorna Wing, Constable, 1971, revised edition 1980. Describes the behaviour of autistic children, and gives practical suggestions for helping them and for coping with family life.

Treatment of Autistic Children, Patricia Howlin and Michael Rutter, Wiley, Chichester, 1987. Practical approaches to the management of problems for families with an autistic child.

Cerebral Palsy

Handling the Young Cerebral Palsied Child at Home, Nancie R. Finnie, Heinemann Medical, London, 1989. Full of information and sensible advice.

The Family and the Handicapped Child: A Study of Cerebral Palsied Children in Their Homes, Sheila Hewett, etc. Allen & Unwin, London, 1970. A survey of 180 families with a child with cerebral palsy aged 9 and under; how they coped and the effect this had on their lives.

Cerebral Palsy: A Practical Guide, Marion Stanton, Optima, London, 1992. Written by the mother of a child with cerebral palsy. Wide-ranging and helpful.

Down's syndrome

Down's Syndrome: A Guide for Parents, Cliff Cunningham, Human Horizons Series, Souvenir Press, 1988. The essential information that parents need, presented in a straightforward, unpatronizing way. The best book I know for parents of a new baby with Down's syndrome.

Down's Syndrome, Richard Newton in conjunction with the Down's Syndrome Association, Optima, London, 1992. A good introduction to medical aspects of Down's syndrome, development, school and adulthood.

Young Children with Down's Syndrome: Their Development, Upbringing, and Effect on Their Families, Janet Carr, Butterworth, for the Institute for Research into Mental and Multiple Handicap, London, 1975. An account of the first four years of life of a group of children with Down's syndrome, and their families.

Down's Syndrome: Children Growing Up, Janet Carr, Cambridge University Press, 1995. The same group, followed up at the ages of 11 and 21.

Appendix 4: Aids and Equipment

Washing

Bathing: Non-slip mats can make the child feel more secure and independent in the bath. Obtainable from any chemist.

Hair washing: Shampoo shields help to prevent shampoo and water from going over the child's face. Obtainable from Heinz Baby Club, Cherry Tree Road, Watford, Hertfordshire WD2 5SH. Tel: 01923 221717. Fax: 01923 244756.
   Non-stinging shampoo: 'No Tears', available from Boots.

Toilet training

Training aids (pants alarms) obtainable from: Enuresis Resource and Information Centre (ERIC), 65 St Michael's Hill, Bristol BS2 8DZ. Tel: 0117 926 4920. Fax: 0117 925 1640.

Toilet seats, to fit the ordinary toilet to make a child-sized seat, obtainable from Heinz Baby Club (see above).

Grow-tall step: To help the child reach the lavatory seat and to rest her feet on when she has got there, obtainable from Heinz Baby Club (see above).

Musical potties: When the child wets in one of these the urine closes an electrical circuit and starts the music playing. Some children seem to love the music, and it also tells you at once that the child has wet (in the right place) so that she can be reinforced immediately. A basic and a super version (complete with chair and detachable wooden support bar in front), prices £15 and £50 respectively, available from: Toys for the Handicapped, 76 Barracks Road, Sandy Lane Industrial Estate, Stourport-on-Severn, Worcestershire DY13 9QB. Tel: 01299 827820. Fax: 01299 827035.

Musical box: Similar in effect but as an independent unit which can be fitted into a potty or used with a toilet bowl insert. Comes with a single- or two-tone alarm and a flashing red light, or with a tune. Prices £36–£43. Obtainable from: Headingley Scientific Services, 45 Westcombe Avenue, Leeds, West Yorkshire LS8 2BS. Tel: 01532 664222.

Eating and table manners

Plastazote tubing: If cutlery handles are too narrow for the child to hold comfortably they can be made thicker with this tubing. It is supplied in four diameters with four different bores and in various lengths, and can be cut to any length required to fit onto utensils, pencils, paint brushes, etc. Obtainable from: Nottingham Rehab Ltd, 17 Ludlow Hill Road, West Bridgford, Nottinghamshire NG2 6HD. Tel: 01159 452345. Fax: 01159 452124.

Non-slip bowl, with suction device to hold it steady, and trainer beakers, obtainable from Heinz Baby Club (see above) or branches of Boots.

Non-slip mats: These help to hold plates and cups steady – alas, they do not prevent them from being hurled. Dycem mats are obtainable from Boots, the Dycem Multi-Activity Mat from Nottingham Rehab Ltd (see above).

Two-handled mugs: Easier for some children to manage than a cup or beaker. Obtainable from most branches of Boots.

Straws: Useful to help a child gain control of her lips and tongue, and just for the fun of using a straw. Plastic, bendable, straws which do not disintegrate as quickly as ordinary ones, can be ordered from Boots, and plastic tubing is available from their wine-making counter.

Pelican bibs: The rigid pocket at the bottom of the bib saves some food from descending to the floor. Small sizes obtainable from branches of Boots or Mothercare. Adult size obtainable from: James Spencer & Co. Ltd, Moor Road Works, Moor Road, Headingley, Leeds, West Yorkshire LS6 4BH. Tel: 01132 785837. Fax: 01132 743956.

Language

See Appendix 3: Helpful books

Play

See Appendix 3: Helpful books

General advice on aids and equipment

The Disabled Living Foundation, 380–384 Harrow Road, London W9 2HU. A mine of information, which they keep constantly up to date. They are a charity, and due to cuts in funding they are currently unable to deal with telephone enquiries, so please write.

Index

READ MORE IN PENGUIN

In every corner of the world, on every subject under the sun, Penguin represents quality and variety – the very best in publishing today.

For complete information about books available from Penguin – including Puffins, Penguin Classics and Arkana – and how to order them, write to us at the appropriate address below. Please note that for copyright reasons the selection of books varies from country to country.

In the United Kingdom: Please write to *Dept. EP, Penguin Books Ltd, Bath Road, Harmondsworth, West Drayton, Middlesex UB7 0DA*

In the United States: Please write to *Consumer Sales, Penguin USA, P.O. Box 999, Dept. 17109, Bergenfield, New Jersey 07621-0120*. VISA and MasterCard holders call 1-800-253-6476 to order Penguin titles

In Canada: Please write to *Penguin Books Canada Ltd, 10 Alcorn Avenue, Suite 300, Toronto, Ontario M4V 3B2*

In Australia: Please write to *Penguin Books Australia Ltd, P.O. Box 257, Ringwood, Victoria 3134*

In New Zealand: Please write to *Penguin Books (NZ) Ltd, Private Bag 102902, North Shore Mail Centre, Auckland 10*

In India: Please write to *Penguin Books India Pvt Ltd, 706 Eros Apartments, 56 Nehru Place, New Delhi 110 019*

In the Netherlands: Please write to *Penguin Books Netherlands bv, Postbus 3507, NL-1001 AH Amsterdam*

In Germany: Please write to *Penguin Books Deutschland GmbH, Metzlerstrasse 26, 60594 Frankfurt am Main*

In Spain: Please write to *Penguin Books S. A., Bravo Murillo 19, 1° B, 28015 Madrid*

In Italy: Please write to *Penguin Italia s.r.l., Via Felice Casati 20, I–20124 Milano*

In France: Please write to *Penguin France S. A., 17 rue Lejeune, F–31000 Toulouse*

In Japan: Please write to *Penguin Books Japan, Ishikiribashi Building, 2–5–4, Suido, Bunkyo-ku, Tokyo 112*

In Greece: Please write to *Penguin Hellas Ltd, Dimocritou 3, GR–106 71 Athens*

In South Africa: Please write to *Longman Penguin Southern Africa (Pty) Ltd, Private Bag X08, Bertsham 2013*

READ MORE IN PENGUIN

WOMEN'S INTEREST

A History of Their Own Bonnie S. Anderson and Judith P. Zinsser
Volumes One and Two

This is an original and path-breaking European history, the first to
approach the past from the perspective of women. 'A richly textured
account that leaves me overwhelmed with admiration for our fore-
mothers' ability to survive with dignity' – *Los Angeles Times Book Review*

Our Bodies, Ourselves Angela Phillips and Jill Rakusen
A Health Book by and for Women   New Edition

'The bible of the women's health movement' – *Guardian*. 'The most
comprehensive guide we've seen for women' – *Woman's World*. 'Every
woman in the country should be issued with a copy free of charge'
– *Mother & Baby*

The Well Woman Handbook Suzy Hayman

Practical and informative, *The Well Woman Handbook* will enable you to
learn more about your body and put the responsibility for its health back
into your own hands.

The Past Is Before Us Sheila Rowbotham

'An extraordinary, readable distillation of what [Sheila Rowbotham] calls
an "account of ideas in the women's movement in Britain" ... This is a
book written from the inside, but with a clarity that recognizes the need to
unravel ideas without abandoning the excitements and frustrations that
every political movement brings with it' – *Sunday Times*

Banishing the Beast Lucy Bland
English Feminism and Sexual Morality 1885–1914

'Fascinating ... Her work is a timely reminder that balancing social
responsibility and individual rights in sexuality and maternity is far from
being a new debate ... This is scholarly history with a contemporary
relevance' – Sheila Rowbotham

READ MORE IN PENGUIN

WOMEN'S INTEREST

Mixed Messages Brigid McConville

Images of breasts – young and naked, sexual and chic – are everywhere. Yet for many women, the form, functions and health of our own breasts remain shrouded in mystery, ignorance – even fear. The consequences of our culture's breast taboos are tragic: Britain's breast-cancer death rate is the highest in the world. 'Lively, gutsy, fast-paced and information-packed' – Sheila Kitzinger

Against Our Will Susan Brownmiller
Men, Women and Rape

Against Our Will sheds a new and blinding light on the tensions that exist between men and women. It was written to give rape its history. Now, as Susan Brownmiller concludes, 'we must deny it a future'. 'Thoughtful, informative and well researched' – *New Statesman & Society*

Women & Self-Esteem
Linda Tschirhart Sanford and Mary Ellen Donovan

'One of the rare self-help books that links inner and outer change into a full circle of revolution. Women will find a friend in its pages – and also a path to changing the world' – Gloria Steinem

Understanding Women Luise Eichenbaum and Susie Orbach

Understanding Women, an expanded version of *Outside In . . . Inside Out*, is a radical appraisal of women's psychological development based on clinical evidence. 'An exciting and thought-provoking book' – *British Journal of Psychiatry*

Psychoanalysis and Feminism Juliet Mitchell

The author of the widely acclaimed *Woman's Estate* here reassesses Freudian psychoanalysis in an attempt to develop an understanding of the psychology of femininity and the ideological oppression of women.

READ MORE IN PENGUIN

A SELECTION OF HEALTH BOOKS

The Kind Food Guide   Audrey Eyton

Audrey Eyton's all-time bestselling *The F-Plan Diet* turned the nation on to fibre-rich food. Now, as the tide turns against factory farming, she provides the guide destined to bring in a new era of eating.

Baby and Child   Penelope Leach

This comprehensive, authoritative and practical handbook is an essential guide, with sections on every stage of the first five years of life.

Woman's Experience of Sex   Sheila Kitzinger

Fully illustrated with photographs and line drawings, this book explores the riches of women's sexuality at every stage of life. 'A book which any mother could confidently pass on to her daughter – and her partner too' – *Sunday Times*

The Effective Way to Stop Drinking   Beauchamp Colclough

Beauchamp Colclough is an international authority on drink dependency, a reformed alcoholic, and living proof that today's decision is tomorrow's freedom. Follow the expert advice contained here, and it will help you give up drinking – for good.

Living with Alzheimer's Disease and Similar Conditions
Dr Gordon Wilcock

This complete and compassionate self-help guide is designed for families and carers (professional or otherwise) faced with the 'living bereavement' of dementia.

Living with Stress
Cary L. Cooper, Rachel D. Cooper and Lynn H. Eaker

Stress leads to more stress, and the authors of this helpful book show why low levels of stress are desirable and how best we can achieve them in today's world. Looking at those most vulnerable, they demonstrate ways of breaking the vicious circle that can ruin lives.

READ MORE IN PENGUIN

A SELECTION OF HEALTH BOOKS

Living with Asthma and Hay Fever   John Donaldson

For the first time, there are now medicines that can prevent asthma attacks from taking place. Based on up-to-date research, this book shows how the majority of sufferers can beat asthma and hay fever to lead full and active lives.

Anorexia Nervosa   R. L. Palmer

Lucid and sympathetic guidance for those who suffer from this disturbing illness and their families and professional helpers, given with a clarity and compassion that will make anorexia more understandable and consequently less frightening for everyone involved.

Medicines: A Guide for Everybody   Peter Parish

The use of any medicine is always a balance of benefits and risks – this book will help the reader understand how to extend the benefits and reduce the risks. Completely revised, it is written in ordinary, accessible language for the layperson, and is also indispensable to anyone involved in health care.

Other People's Children   Sheila Kitzinger

Though step-families are common, adults and children in this situation often feel isolated because they fail to conform to society's idealized picture of a normal family. This sensitive, incisive book is essential reading for anyone involved with or in a step-family.

Miscarriage   Ann Oakley, Ann McPherson and Helen Roberts

One million women worldwide become pregnant every day. At least half of these pregnancies end in miscarriage or stillbirth. But each miscarriage is the loss of a potential baby, and that loss can be painful to adjust to. Here is sympathetic support and up-to-date information on one of the commonest areas of women's reproductive experience.

READ MORE IN PENGUIN

A SELECTION OF HEALTH BOOKS

When a Woman's Body Says No to Sex   Linda Valins

Vaginismus – an involuntary spasm of the vaginal muscles that prevents penetration – has been discussed so little that many women who suffer from it don't recognize their condition by its name. Linda Valins's practical and compassionate guide will liberate these women from their fears and sense of isolation and help them find the right form of therapy.

Mixed Messages   Brigid McConville

Images of breasts – young and naked, sexual and chic – are everywhere. Yet for many women, the form, functions and health of our own breasts remain shrouded in mystery, ignorance – even fear. The consequences of our culture's breast taboos are tragic: Britain's breast-cancer death rate is the highest in the world. Every woman should read *Mixed Messages* – the first book to consider the well-being of our breasts in the wider contexts of our lives.

Defeating Depression   Tony Lake

Counselling, medication, and the support of friends can all provide invaluable help in relieving depression. But if we are to combat it once and for all, we must face up to perhaps painful truths about our past and take the first steps forward that can eventually transform our lives. This lucid and sensitive book shows us how.

Freedom and Choice in Childbirth   Sheila Kitzinger

Undogmatic, honest and compassionate, Sheila Kitzinger's book raises searching questions about the kind of care offered to the pregnant woman – and will help her make decisions and communicate effectively about the kind of birth experience she desires.

The Complete New Herbal   Richard Mabey

The new bible for herb users – authoritative, up-to-date, absorbing to read and hugely informative, with practical, clear sections on cultivation and the uses of herbs in daily life, nutrition and healing.

READ MORE IN PENGUIN

A SELECTION OF HEALTH BOOKS

Twins, Triplets and More Elizabeth Bryan

This enlightening study of the multiple birth phenomenon covers all aspects of the subject from conception and birth to old age and death. It also offers much comfort and support as well as carefully researched information gained from meeting several thousands of children and their families.

Meditation for Everybody Louis Proto

Meditation means liberation from stress, anxiety and depression. This lucid and readable book by the author of *Self-Healing* describes a variety of meditative practices. From simple breathing exercises to more advanced techniques, there is something here to suit everybody's needs.

Endometriosis Suzie Hayman

Endometriosis is currently surrounded by many damaging myths. Suzie Hayman's pioneering book will set the record straight and provide both sufferers and their doctors with the information necessary for an improved understanding of this frequently puzzling condition.

The New Our Bodies, Ourselves
The Boston Women's Health Book Collective

To be used by all generations, *The New Our Bodies, Ourselves* courageously discusses many difficult issues, and is tailored to the needs of women in the 1990s. It provides the most complete advice and information available on women's health care. This British edition is by Angela Phillips and Jill Rakusen.

Not On Your Own Sally Burningham
The MIND Guide to Mental Health

Cutting through the jargon and confusion surrounding the subject of mental health to provide clear explanations and useful information, *Not On Your Own* will enable those with problems – as well as their friends and relatives – to make the best use of available help or find their own ways to cope.

READ MORE IN PENGUIN

A CHOICE OF NON-FICTION

The Time of My Life Denis Healey

'Denis Healey's memoirs have been rightly hailed for their intelligence, wit and charm ... *The Time of My Life* should be read, certainly for pleasure, but also for profit ... he bestrides the post war world, a Colossus of a kind' – *Independent*. 'No finer autobiography has been written by a British politician this century' – *Economist*

Far Flung Floyd Keith Floyd

Keith Floyd's latest culinary odyssey takes him to the far flung East and the exotic flavours of Malaysia, Hong Kong, Vietnam and Thailand. The irrepressible Floyd as usual spices his recipes with witty stories, wry observation and a generous pinch of gastronomic wisdom.

Genie Russ Rymer

In 1970 thirteen-year-old Genie emerged from a terrible captivity. Her entire childhood had been spent in one room, caged in a cot or strapped in a chair. Almost mute, without linguistic or social skills, Genie aroused enormous excitement among the scientists who took over her life. 'Moving and terrifying ... opens windows some might prefer kept shut on man's inhumanity' – Ruth Rendell

The Galapagos Affair John Treherne

Stories about Friedrich Ritter and Dore Strauch, settlers on the remote Galapagos island of Floreana, quickly captivated the world's press in the early thirties. Then death and disappearance took the rumours to fever pitch ... 'A tale of brilliant mystery' – Paul Theroux

1914 Lyn Macdonald

'Once again she has collected an extraordinary mass of original accounts, some by old soldiers, some in the form of diaries and journals, even by French civilians ... Lyn Macdonald's research has been vast, and in result is triumphant' – Raleigh Trevelyan in the *Tablet*. 'These poignant voices from the past conjure up a lost innocence as well as a lost generation' – *Mail on Sunday*